100
Short Cases
for the
MRCP

100
Short Cases
for the
MRCP

Second edition

K. Gupta
MBBS, MRCP, FACP
Professor of Clinical Medicine
New York Medical College
Valhalla, NY, USA

Consulting editors

P. Carmichael
BSc, MB, BCh, MRCP
MRC Research Fellow
Department of Nephrology
Royal Free Hospital
London, UK

and

A. Zumla
BSc, MB, ChB, MSc, MRCP, PhD
Associate Professor
Center for Infectious Diseases
University of Texas Medical School and School of Public Health
Houston, USA

(former Senior Registrar, Departments of Immunology and
Medicine, Royal Postgraduate Medical School, Hammersmith
Hospital, London, UK)

CHAPMAN & HALL MEDICAL
London · Glasgow · Weinheim · New York · Tokyo · Melbourne · Madras

Published by Chapman & Hall, 2–6 Boundary Row, London SE1 8HN, UK

Chapman & Hall, 2–6 Boundary Row, London SE1 8HN, UK

Blackie Academic & Professional, Wester Cleddens Road, Bishopbriggs, Glasgow G64 2NZ, UK

Chapman & Hall GmbH, Pappelallee 3, 69469 Weinheim, Germany

Chapman & Hall USA, One Penn Plaza, 41st Floor, New York NY 10119, USA

Chapman & Hall Japan, ITP-Japan, Kyowa Building, 3F, 2-2-1 Hirakawacho, Chiyoda-ku, Tokyo 102, Japan

Chapman & Hall Australia, Thomas Nelson Australia, 102 Dodds Street, South Melbourne, Victoria 3205, Australia

Chapman & Hall India, R. Seshadri, 32 Second Main Road, CIT East, Madras 600 035, India

First edition 1983

Reprinted 1984, 1986, 1987, 1991

Second edition 1994

© 1994 K. Gupta

Typeset in 10/12pt Palatino by Mews Photosetting, Beckenham, Kent

Printed in Great Britain by St Edmundsbury Press, Bury St Edmunds

ISBN 0 412 54860 7

A catalogue record for this book is available from the British Library

Library of Congress Catalog Card Number 94-71816

∞ Printed on permanent acid-free text paper, manufactured in accordance with the proposed ANSI/NISO Z39.48-1992 and ANSI/NISO Z39.48-1984 (Permanence of Paper).

Contents

Foreword

The purpose of the clinical part of the examination for the membership diploma of the Royal College of Physicians (UK) is to ensure that successful candidates have acquired a high standard of history taking and physical examination, and are capable of sound judgement in interpreting their findings, in advancing sensible differential diagnoses and in planning investigations and management, taking into consideration all physical, psychological and social factors. The achievement of this high standard depends greatly on the depth and breadth of the candidate's experience at the bedside and in the clinic, and on the responsibility which he has held for making important clinical decisions under the general guidance of a senior physician. Experience of this kind sharpens the clinical acumen of the trainee physician and engenders in him a disciplined routine of physical examination which he can appropriately modify to deal with a wide spectrum of clinical patterns of disease. The presentation of 'short cases' in the clinical part of the MRCP examination specifically concentrates on this aspect of training.

This little book is intended to heighten the candidate's awareness of commonly encountered clinical patterns of abnormal physical signs and to draw his attention to the kind of questions he should be repeatedly asking himself as the pattern unfolds before him. Hopefully, it will stimulate within him a freer association of ideas, which he can then proceed to test further as his physical examination proceeds. The book makes no attempt to be comprehensive. It understandably centres upon the more commonly encountered patterns of physical signs in clinical practice in the United Kingdom and upon a number of rarer conditions which have traditionally been selected for examinations because they present with striking physical signs. The aspiring candidate for the membership would do well to browse through this book and to annotate and expand upon it in ways related to his own personal experiences. He would also be well advised to ask a senior colleague to observe him in action when presented with a variety of 'short cases' and so discover whether he has learnt his lesson and developed a comprehensive, efficient and imaginative approach to each problem.

This book is clearly the product of an author who, together with his advisers, has been subjected to the rigours of the MRCP clinical examination, and I am confident that the advice contained herein will be of inestimable value to those who follow in his footsteps.

J.M. Ledingham
MD FRCP
Emeritus Professor of Medicine

Note: in this book the personal pronouns 'he' and 'she' are used interchangeably unless otherwise specified.

Preface

By the time a candidate sits for Part II of the MRCP examination, he or she will have acquired a good theoretical knowledge of medicine, along with practical experience of dealing with a significant number of patients while working as a junior hospital doctor. Most British examinations for higher diplomas, in particular the MRCP, are well known for the considerable importance they attach to the clinical section of the examination: to fail this part of the examination is to fail the whole examination. Most candidates find the 'short cases' more difficult to pass than the 'long case', where the candidate has a full 60 minutes at his or her disposal. In a non-examination situation, such as day-to-day hospital practice, one is relatively at ease, with plenty of time to examine the patient, take a good history and at times to check and recheck, say, the presence or absence of a particular heart murmur or hepatic or splenic enlargement. This is not the case under examination conditions, where the candidate is being watched constantly by two examiners and can be overcome with fear of failure. Not surprisingly, this puts extra pressure on the candidate, who is usually expected (without enquiring about the patient's symptoms) not only to carry out the physical examination in an established fashion, but to correlate the relevant findings and present a short case report in a limited period of 3–5 minutes. In 30 minutes, the candidate is expected to examine as many as six to eight short cases. Speed and thoroughness in physical examination are vital in arriving at a sensible, probable diagnosis.

The continuing success of this handbook, originally published some 10 years ago, has resulted in this second edition. New material has been added to almost all the short cases.

Every attempt has been made to maintain the unique approach to the short cases based on what is required in the examination setting. This book must be considered only as a supplement to your fundamental knowledge and the clinical experience acquired through years of interaction with hundreds, if not thousands, of patients. It is certainly not meant to be a comprehensive textbook of medicine or physical signs. In fact, my intention is to maintain this work as a handbook that graduate and postgraduate students can easily carry in their pockets.

This book is intended mainly to help final MRCP candidates. The goal is to enable them to develop a methodical, accurate and comprehensive approach to the commonly given short cases so that they can avoid repeated half-hearted demonstrations of physical signs. Besides the MRCP, the book should be great help for qualifying examinations in medicine and other postgraduate qualifications that are equivalent to MRCP, such as FRACP (Australia and New Zealand), FCP (South Africa) and MD (India).

K. Gupta
MB, MRCP (UK)

Acknowledgements

I am most appreciative of the encouragement and suggestions of Mr Paul Remes, Senior Editor, Chapman & Hall, without whom this second edition would not have been possible. My thanks are due to numerous physicians, students and hundreds of MRCP candidates for their constructive criticism and praise for this book. Finally, I am thankful to my wife, Dr Veena Gupta MD MRCOG (London) and children for their time and tolerance during my continued involvement in over a dozen books including this second edition.

K. Gupta

Introduction

WHAT ARE EXAMINERS LOOKING FOR?

Examining MRCP candidates on short cases remains a unique way of testing the clinical skills of the aspiring physician who can be considered as 'consultant material'. At least for general internal medicine, MRCP with its high standard (together with its high failure rate) remains one of the most challenging tests of clinical skills in the world. Although one is expected to pass separately in all three sections (the written, oral and clinical examinations), most candidates find the clinical examination to be a major hurdle. The clinical examination itself consists of a 'long' case and the short cases. The short cases have a higher failure rate (higher mortality) than the long case. The examiners are particularly interested in assessing whether or not the candidate can accomplish the following:

A. Can satisfactorily elicit physical signs in a given patient with confidence.
B. Based on physical findings locally, is able to think and look for relevant physical signs elsewhere (for example, in a patient with ascites looking for other stigmata of cirrhosis).
C. Can come up with the most likely diagnosis and the other two or three close conditions, the differential diagnosis. Most experienced examiners are interested in your interpretation of the physical findings and not in the precise diagnosis.
D. Has acquired the competency in planning the relevant investigations and treatment modalities for some of the common clinical conditions.

Besides the above aspects, the examiners can easily judge your knowledge of aetiology, pathophysiology and complications, etc. through the use of common questions and brief answers.

HOW TO IMPROVE YOUR SKILLS FOR SHORT CASES

In order to acquire the speed and thoroughness necessary for passing the short cases, the following steps have been noted to be helpful by hundreds of those who have successfully passed the MRCP examination:

1. Clinical medicine can only be learned through sound clinical practice and experience. Remember that there are no short cuts when it comes to learning clinical skills. Try to enhance your ability to elicit physical signs through frequent critical evaluation by a senior colleague. Having the other 2–3 MRCP candidates watch your technique of physical examination can be extremely helpful. Attending the MRCP courses can also gear you up for the exams. Many otherwise brilliant candidates fail the finals simply because of a lack of practice and inability to comprehend the rules of MRCP examination.
2. Develop a list of short cases. The hundred most common short cases are already here in this book. For each short case, think of a plan of systematic examination; a haphazard technique of examination can only ensure failure.
3. Always think in terms of what you are looking for in the area of examination (locally) and then quickly look for other relevant physical signs (elsewhere). This is the approach that has been adopted for all short cases described in this book.
4. Put the physical findings together and quickly come up with the most likely diagnosis.
5. Think of the other two or three close conditions, the differential diagnosis. Remember the golden rule – common conditions are common and rare conditions rare. Don't commit the mistake of giving 13 differential diagnoses

and possibilities for each short case; the examiners can easily detect that your knowledge is more theoretical than practical.

6. Do not spend all your time just on one or two cases. Remember, you are expected to see several short cases during this limited time. If you are unable to make a diagnosis, that is fine. Give your positive findings and the most likely diagnosis. A candidate who is able to cover 5–7 short cases and gets 1 wrong has a better chance of success than someone who is slow and is able to see only 2–3 cases and still gets 1 wrong!

7. As you will note from the presentation in this book, it is important to develop a list of 3–4 important questions for each short case. The examiners are interested in assessing your basic knowledge of a particular condition through these questions.

8. While discussing the investigations, do not jump at the most sophisticated and expensive method of investigation. In most cases, CT scan and MRI investigations should come up in your discussion only after the simpler and more common investigations (blood, urine, stool tests, etc.) have been covered.

9. While discussing the treatment, always think in terms of non-pharmacological treatment first (for example, weight loss, physical exercise and other lifestyle changes for hypertension, diabetes and coronary heart disease, etc.). Try to discuss the treatment under appropriate medical and surgical categories if applicable.

10. Do not try to impress the examiner with your knowledge of a new diagnosis or treatment approach that you read about only last week in the *British Medical Journal* or the *Lancet*. Take a stepwise approach and first discuss the conventional and well-established principles of diagnosis and management. The examiner may not have had a chance to catch up with his own last week's *BMJ* or *Lancet*!

PART 1

Looking at the Patient

GENERAL ADVICE

It is polite and appropriate for you to introduce yourself to the patient and tell the patient that you would like to examine him/her.

The following cases are very common in the short case section of the MRCP exam and test the skills of the candidate at recognizing abnormal physical signs and following them up to look for signs locally and elsewhere to make a diagnosis or come up with reasonable differential diagnoses. Do not spend too much time on these cases.

Listen to the examiner's instructions very carefully. Usually the instructions are very explicit and clear. Candidates should not get onto the wrong track by not following the stated instructions. If you are not sure what the examiner's request is, ask him/her for a clarification. For example, in a case of acromegaly if the examiner says to you 'Look at the patient's face and tell me the diagnosis', the diagnosis will be obvious to you so tell the examiner that you think the patient has features of acromegaly and would like to examine him/her further for other signs. However, if the examiner says 'Look at the patient's face and then go on to examine him appropriately', then the instructions should allow you to proceed to look for other signs of acromegaly.

Most of the 'look at the patient' cases involve easy spot diagnosis and the examiner will be assessing your skills at eliciting physical signs and looking for other features of the condition.

Once you have identified the clue to the diagnosis, you then have to go on to elicit all the physical signs associated with that particular condition, firstly by continuing with examination of the face and then looking for other features of the condition elsewhere.

If, after you have completed the physical examination, you are not sure of the diagnosis, do not lose hope. Just go on to present your findings confidently and try out a differential diagnosis. The examiner might help drag the diagnosis out of you.

CASE 1 PAGETOID SKULL

Examiner

Look at this elderly man's face and tell me what you see.

Locally (relevant features)

- Distinctive box-like enlargement of the skull.
- Palpate the scalp for an irregular (corrugated) surface.
- Hearing impairment; note presence of hearing aid or deafness of patient on introducing yourself.

Elsewhere (to confirm your suspicions or to get supportive signs)

- Look for convex bowing and/or lateral bowing of tibial and femoral bones respectively.
- Look for signs of high output cardiac failure.
- Examine the fundi for angioid streaks.

Candidate

This patient has Paget's disease characterized by ... (go on to give your physical findings).

Examiner

What investigations would you ask for in this patient?

Candidate

1. X-ray of the skull (lucent cortical infarctions and areas of bone resorption and new bone formation).
2. Serum calcium, phosphate and alkaline phosphatase.
3. Technetium ^{99}m diphosphonate bone scan.

Examiner

What are the three most common complications, assuming disease elsewhere?

Candidate

1. Pathological fracture.
2. Neurological complications, e.g. nerve deafness, platybasia, spinal cord compression.
3. High output cardiac failure.

Other complications:

- Osteogenic sarcoma (1%).
- Nephrolithiasis.
- Hypercalcaemia.

Examiner

What treatment is available?

Candidate

Most patients require no treatment. Bone pain may be controlled by simple analgesics (aspirin/non-steroidal). More severe cases may require the use of alternative drugs. Those commonly used are: diphosphonates, calcitonin (salmon or porcine), sodium fluoride, actinomycin-D. Treatment of complications involves treatment of neural compression, high output cardiac failure, repeated fractures and hypercalcaemia.

Discussion on Paget's disease

Paget's disease of the bone is most commonly seen in people of West European origin, it is a rare condition in the Indian sub-continent, China, Japan, the Middle East, and interestingly, Scandinavia. In the UK and USA, it affects approximately 3% of the population over the age of 40 and there is no sex preference. The aetiology remains undefined although a viral aetiology has been suggested and an association with nucleocapsids of measle-like viruses has been described. Clinically, most patients are asymptomatic with the mono-ostotic variety predominating.

The bones characteristically affected by the disease include the skull, spine, pelvis, femur, tibia, clavicle and humerus. Initial presentation is often pain in the affected bone. Biochemically, the serum calcium and phosphate levels are normal with an elevated alkaline phosphatase. Radiologically, the affected bone often shows expansion with loss of cortical definition and replacement of the normally well demarcated cortex and medulla by a coarse, striated pattern often denser than normal. Remodelling often follows the lines of stress, thus, the weight bearing bones (femur and tibia) tend to become bowed.

CASE 2 ACROMEGALY

Examiner

Look at this man's face and tell me what the diagnosis is.

Be sensitive to what you say in front of the patient.

Locally

- Prognathism (protruding lower jaw – bottom set of teeth overriding the upper set).
- General coarseness of facial features.
- Macroglossia (ask patient to stick tongue out).
- Large lips, nose and ear lobes, plus a long face.

Elsewhere

- Glance at the large hands with sausage shaped fingers.
- Examine palms for increased sweating.
- Look for features of carpal tunnel syndrome.

Candidate

This patient has clinical features of acromegaly . . . (then go on to give your physical findings).

Examiner

Is there anything that you would like to ask the patient?

Candidate

I have five questions:

1. Have you or any member of your family noted any change in your facial appearance over the past couple of years?
2. Have you had recent changes in the size of the clothes, gloves, shoes?
3. Do you suffer from headaches?

4. Have you noticed any increased problems with sweating?
5. Have you had any problems with vision?

Examiner

What investigations would you request?

Candidate

- Serum fasting growth hormone level, plus its value during an oral glucose tolerance test (OGTT).
- Assess the patient's visual field.
- Lateral skull X-ray, CT scan/MRI scan of pituitary fossa.
- Fasting glucose plus an OGTT.
- Make an assessment of the rest of pituitary function, e.g. measure the levels of TSH and FSH/LH, plus an insulin tolerance test to assess the competency of the hypothalamic-adrenocortical axis.
- Heel pad thickness as measured radiologically, greater than 18 mm in women and 21 mm in men is regarded as confirmatory.

Examiner

Does this patient have active acromegaly?

Candidate

His palms were moist and sweaty and this may be indicative of disease activity.

Examiner

What treatments are available for this condition?

Candidate

- Transsphenoidal pituitary surgery.
- Pituitary irradiation.
- Adjunctive therapy using bromocriptine.

Discussion on acromegaly

Acromegaly results from excessive production of growth hormone from a pituitary adenoma. It most frequently occurs in middle age with a prevalence of 30 to 50 per million of the population. Associated conditions include hypertension (20–30%), diabetes mellitus (12%), impaired glucose tolerance (25%), and a diffuse or nodular goitre (20%). Almost 50% of non-hypertensive acromegalics have a cardiomyopathy, explaining the increased incidence of cardiac failure found in this condition. If untreated, signs and symptoms of hypopituitarism may develop. Acromegaly may occur as part of a polyendocrine syndrome referred to as multiple endocrine adenomatosis (MEA) type 1 (Werner's syndrome) which is characterized by the occurrence of tumours producing peptide hormones in the parathyroid, pituitary and pancreatic glands simultaneously. It is inherited in an autosomal dominant fashion.

CASE 3 HYDROCEPHALUS

Examiner

Look at this man's face and tell me what you see.

Locally

- Note the globular, smooth and symmetrically enlarged skull.
- The eyeballs are prominent and are pushed downwards so that the upper part of the sclera is visible.
- Examine the eyes for papilloedema or optic atrophy (sometimes patients with 'normal pressure hydrocephalus' appear in the exam).

Candidate

The most striking feature is that this man's head appears to be disproportionately large. In particular, he has a symmetrically enlarged smooth skull, with normal facial bones and mildly proptosed eyes.

Examiner

What is your differential diagnosis?

Candidate

- Paget's disease of the skull.
- Achondroplasia; relative to the small body the head is disproportionately large.
- Soto's syndrome; or cerebral gigantism, an autosomal dominant condition consisting of macrocephaly, a triangular face, mental slowness and macrosomia.
- Frontal bossing of sickle cell anaemia.

Examiner

What do you understand by the term 'normal pressure hydrocephalus'?

Candidate

This is a syndrome of communicating hydrocephalus with normal intracranial pressure which often presents in the elderly, with gait ataxia, dementia and urinary incontinence. The cerebrospinal fluid pressure is normal. The majority of patients respond to ventricular shunting. The precise aetiology remains unknown.

Discussion on hydrocephalus

Hydrocephalus may be divided into non-communicating and communicating types.

Non-communicating hydrocephalus occurs when cerebrospinal fluid escape from the fourth ventricle is obstructed. This may develop as a result of a number of developmental abnormalities, such as aqueductal stenosis, the Dandy-Walker malformation and the various Chiari malformations. Additional causes include neoplasms and cysts located either within the ventricular system or impinging on structures in the posterior fossa. These must be looked for.

Communicating hydrocephalus, where the cerebrospinal fluid escape into the fourth ventricle is not totally impaired, tends to develop as a result of meningeal scarring after infection or intraventricular haemorrhage in the perinatal period, with resultant leptomeningeal scarring.

CASE 4 HYPERTHYROIDISM

Examiner

I want you to look at this woman's face and then examine her appropriately.

Locally

- To help one to focus on the potential causes, it should be taken into consideration that you are looking at a young woman. Thus, one should consider: nerve lesions (should be obvious); endocrine disorders; autoimmune conditions; and dermatological conditions.
- In this case, one should be struck by the staring look of the patient, due to her exophthalmos and lid retraction.
- Note whether the exophthalmos is unilateral, bilateral, and if bilateral whether it is symmetrical on both sides or not.
- Lid lag should then be formally examined for (with your finger two feet away, request the patient to follow your finger with her eyes as you move it from a position of maximum elevation downwards. The upper eyelid lags behind the cornea in moving down and thus more of the sclera is exposed).
- Exophthalmos is better seen from the lateral side or from above the patient's head.
- Test for diplopia since myopathy of the eye muscles may be present.

Elsewhere

- Look for fine tremor of the outstretched hands.
- Look for thyroid acropachy (clubbing-like changes).
- Examine for tachycardia.
- Shake hands and feel for warm sweaty palms.
- Look/palpate for a goitre; if present, listen for a bruit.

Additional features

Look for pretibial myxoedema over the shins.

- Look for thyrotoxic myopathy (shoulder muscle wasting).
- Examine skin for vitiligo.

Examiner

Assuming that the aetiology here is that of Grave's disease, what would your treatment strategy be?

Candidate

In view of the fact that this is a woman who still wishes to have a family, her thyrotoxic state should be first controlled using beta blockers and carbimazole, and then she should be referred to the surgeons for a partial thyroidectomy.

Examiner

What do you understand by the term 'sick euthyroid'?

Candidate

This is a condition involving alterations in the peripheral transport and/or metabolism of thyroid hormones with or without alterations in their central regulation. Reduced production of T_3 due to inhibition of the peripheral 5'-monodeiodination of T_4 is a consistent feature of this syndrome. It occurs in the setting of a severe illness or physical trauma. Patients generally remain euthyroid except those who are severely ill, when serum total and free levels of T_4 and T_3 fall with an inadequate compensatory rise in TSH. The high levels of rT_3 distinguish this condition from pituitary hypothyroidism. However, the metabolic impact of sick euthyroid syndrome on peripheral tissues remains unclear, as does the need for thyroid hormone treatment.

Examiner

What is T_3 thyrotoxicosis?

Candidate

This is a form of thyrotoxicosis where patients have normal levels of plasma T_4 (thyroxine) but raised T_3 (triiodothyronine) levels. The clinical features are the same as those of T_4 excess.

Examiner

What is pretibial myxoedema?

Candidate

This is the term given to thickened, raised plaques of skin with 'peau d'orange' appearance over the dorsum of the legs or feet which occur in cases of untreated hyperthyroidism. Since they are usually found over the shins they are called 'pretibial myxoedema'.

Discussion on hyperthyrodism

Note that there may be questions on 'struma ovarii' which is a source of ectopic thyroid stimulating hormone (TSH) and thus an abdominal ultrasound would feature in your investigations in discussion on this subject.

Choriocarcinoma may also be a source of ectopic TSH and thus a pregnancy test or HCG levels would feature in your list of investigations.

CASE 5 HYPOTHYROIDISM

Examiner

Look at this patient's face and tell me what you think the diagnosis might be.

Locally

- Note the coarse facial features; dry thickened skin, puffiness around the eyelids.
- Feel the sparse, coarse hair.
- Assess the patient's speech (ask the address): speech is slow, monotonous and the voice is hoarse and croaky.
- Look at the tongue for macroglossia.

Elsewhere

- Look for:

  - Bradycardia.
  - Rough dry skin.
  - Slow relaxation of the ankle jerk.
  - Scar of previous thyroidectomy.
  - Carpal tunnel syndrome (see Case 83).
  - Deafness.

Candidate

This patient has an expressionless face with general puffiness, especially peri-orbitally. His skin is coarse and dry (touch it), with thin, lacklustre hair. His speech is slow, monotonous and hoarse (assess by asking him what his name is and where he lives) and I note that he has an old thyroidectomy scar. He most probably suffers from hypothyroidism, and to confirm this clinically I would wish to check his pulse for bradycardia and his ankle jerks for delayed relaxation. A possible alternative diagnosis is that of depression.

Examiner

What are the causes of hypothyroidism?

Candidate

The common causes of hypothyroidism are:

1. Chronic autoimmune thyroiditis (Hashimoto's thyroiditis).
2. Post surgical resection or radio-iodine therapy for hyperthyroidism.
3. Secondary to anti-thyroid drugs, e.g. carbimazole, etc.

Other causes include:

- Diet with endemic goitre.
- Developmental abnormalities, e.g. agenesis and mal-development.
- Dyshormonogenesis.
- Hypopituitarism.

Examiner

What are the neuropsychiatric manifestations that may be found in this condition?

Candidate

These include:

1. Neurological:
   a. Hearing deficit.
   b. Carpal tunnel syndrome.
   c. Polyneuropathy.
   d. Cerebellar dysfunction.
   e. Diminished deep tendon reflexes.
2. Psychiatric:
   a. Mental obtundness.
   b. Mimicking dementia.
   c. Depression
   d. Paranoia.

Examiner

What one question would you like to ask this patient?

Candidate

Which weather do you prefer: hot or cold? Patients with myxoedema prefer hot weather.

CASE 6 CUSHING'S SYNDROME

Examiner

Look at this woman and tell me what your diagnosis is, and why.

Locally

- Note the 'moon'-shaped rounded face with plethoric appearance which gives you the clue to the diagnosis.
- Note the acne and hirsutism.
- Look for conjunctival oedema and crinkly skin (gently pinch the forearm skin).

Elsewhere

- Examine for 'buffalo hump'.
- Truncal obesity.
- Look for purple striae over the abdomen.
- Purpura and spontaneous bruising may be present over the limbs.
- Request permission to examine blood pressure (may have hypertension).
- Test for myopathy if examiner allows.

Candidate

This middle-aged lady is somewhat obese, the distribution of which is predominantly truncal and facial in nature. She has a phlethoric complexion, is somewhat hirsute and displays cervical and supraclavicular (if exposed) fat pads. This constellation of signs together with her axillary striae and forearm bruising make me think that the diagnosis is that of Cushing's syndrome.

Examiner

Is there anything else that you would wish to do?

Candidate

Yes, I would like to measure her BP, as most patients with this condition are hypertensive due to fluid and salt retention secondary to the excess corticosteroids. If a urine sample was available I would dip stick test it for glucose.

Examiner

What investigations would you ask for?

Candidate

Investigations should be directed towards:

1. Confirming the clinical suspicion of excessive corticosteroid production.
2. Determining the cause of the abnormality.

Thus, I would ask for: urinary free cortisols, as this gives an approximate indication of cortisol production, and, if these are elevated, a 24-hour urinary collection for cortisol should then be performed. Supportive dynamic tests include:

– 'Low dose dexamethasone test'.
– 'Insulin tolerance test'.

The former induces a fall in the serum cortisol and the latter induces a rise in normal individuals. The converse is the finding in patients with Cushing's syndrome. Documenting the abolition of the circadian rhythm is also confirmatory, though it has to be performed on an in-patient basis. To establish the cause, the plasma ACTH level should be measured, and additionally metyrapone and high dose dexamethasone tests performed. A high level of plasma ACTH will imply an ectopic source which would then require a malignancy screen. An excessive response to metyrapone, i.e. a marked increase in precortisol metabolites, would imply a pituitary source, as would the suppressibility of serum cortisol in a high dose dexamethasone test. Radiological studies should then be directed to the appropriate organ(s).

Examiner

What do you understand by the term Nelson's syndrome?

Candidate

Nelson's syndrome formerly occurred as a complication of bilateral adrenalectomy for Cushing's disease. Over a 10-year period 10% to 20% of patients treated in this way will develop the syndrome. This is now less common due to the treatment of choice now being surgical resection of the pituitary adenoma by the trans-sphenoidal approach. The mechanism is very straightforward: in the absence of the negative feedback effect of cortisol, the ACTH secreting pituitary adenoma expands, causing headaches, visual problems and, if not treated, hypopituitarism. The characteristic increased pigmentation is secondary to a melanocyte stimulating component of the ACTH precursor molecule, pro-opiomelanocortin. In cases where an adenoma is not radiologically demonstrable, exploration of the pituitary fossa with or without venous sampling is carried out in those patients with a positive high dose dexamethasone suppression test. If no adenoma is found, a hypophysectomy is often performed. In those centres where bilateral adrenalectomy is performed in the absence of pituitary irradiation, then over a period of time a proportion may develop Nelson's syndrome.

Discussion on Cushing's syndrome

The term Cushing's syndrome is used to describe the clinical disorder that results from supraphysiological levels of corticosteroids in the circulation. It may vary in severity in an individual patient, and spontaneous remissions or cyclical recurrences occasionally occur. For convenience, the syndrome may be divided into two broad categories, namely: ACTH dependent and non-ACTH dependent.

1. ACTH dependent causes:
   a. Pituitary-dependent bilateral adrenocortical hyperplasia (Cushing's disease).

    b. Ectopic ACTH syndrome.
    c. Iatrogenic.
2. Non-ACTH dependent causes:
    a. Adenomas/carcinomas of the adrenal cortex.
    b. Iatrogenic (cause is common, being a manifestation of the widespread use of steroids as a therapeutic tool).

Excluding iatrogenic and ectopic causes, approximately 80% of cases are due to Cushing's disease, which has a female predominance of 8:1, with the remaining 20% being equally divided between adenomas and carcinomas of the adrenal gland.

CASE 7 ACHONDROPLASIA

Examiner

From what condition does this patient suffer?

Locally

- Skull appears enlarged but this is because of the short stature rather than true increase in skull size.
- The forehead is prominent and bulging.
- The saddle nose (depressed nose bridge) is obvious.

Elsewhere

- Make the patient stand and measure height (short); note gross shortening of all four limbs but a normal trunk length.
- Note that dorsal kyphosis with lumbar lordosis is present.
- The hands are small with the fingers being almost of equal length.

Candidate

This gentleman suffers from dwarfism. Due to the disproportionate shortening of his four limbs in relation to his skull and trunk, the most likely diagnosis is that of achondroplasia which is inherited in an autosomal dominant fashion.

Examiner

What other forms of dwarfism do you know of?

Candidate

Other forms include those due to:

1. Developmental deficiencies of endocrine hormones such as growth hormone (Laron dwarfism), and thyroid hormone (cretinism).

2. Excessive hormones may also have an equally deleterious effect during development, such as cortisol (Cushing's syndrome).
3. Less common causes of small stature include gonadal dysgenesis and pseudohypopituitarism.

Discussion on achondroplasia

Achondroplasia is an autosomal dominant condition and is characterized by a defective cartilaginous growth plate. Affected individuals nevertheless have normal mental and sexual functions and there is no shortening of the lifespan. They are normal sexually too.

CASE 8 KLINEFELTER'S SYNDROME
(47XXY or 46XY/47XXY)

Examiner

From what genetic condition does this man suffer?

Striking features

- Tall patient with disproportionately long lower limbs gives a clue to the diagnosis.
- Look for gynaecomastia (50% of cases).
- Examine axillary and facial hair: these are absent/sparse.
- May have obesity and varicose veins.

Candidate

The most likely diagnosis is that of Klinefelter's syndrome; there is tallness of stature with disproportionately long legs, gynaecomastia and obesity. Normally, I would also examine this man's testicles which I would expect to be shrunken and firm.

Examiner

Are such men fertile?

Candidate

No, they are infertile being azoospermic due to a lack of germ cells within the testes which tend to be hyalinized.

Examiner

What are the potential karyotypes that this man could have?

Candidate

Such a condition is due to at least one extra X chromosome,

90% of affected individuals being 47XXY (or more than two X) with the remaining 10% being mosaics 46XY/47XXY.

Discussion on Klinefelter's syndrome

Klinefelter's syndrome is the most common cause of male hypogonadism, affecting 1:500 males. The diagnosis is made with a buccal smear for karyotype analysis. Plasma gonadotropin levels are increased. The incidence increases with advancing maternal and paternal age. With increasing numbers of X chromosomes, the incidence of mental retardation increases. There is an increased risk of breast cancer, i.e. twenty times that of normal males, though still only a fifth of that found in women. The mosaic form (46XY/47XXY) tends to be less severe in all respects, often with normal testes and, occasionally, fertility. Many of these patients are also obese and have an increased incidence of disorders such as diabetes, bronchiectasis and varicose veins.

CASE 9 DOWN'S SYNDROME

Examiner

What is the most likely condition that this young man has?

Locally

Facial features:

- Note small stature with low set ears.
- Face is expressionless and the skull small.
- Eyes are slanted and epicanthal folds are present.

The above three will give you a clue as to the diagnosis and you should then focus on examining the patient for Down's syndrome signs.

- Examine the eyes for a convergent squint and Brushfield's spots (grey/white specks of depigmentation on the periphery of the iris). Lens opacities may be present.
- Flat bridge of the nose will be apparent.
- Tongue is rather large, protruding and fissured.

Elsewhere

- Examine the hands:
  - Short and broad.
  - Single palmar crease.
  - Fingers are small.
  - Little finger is incurved (clinodactyly) with an ulnar convexity.
  - An absent second phalanx in the little finger.

Candidate

This gentleman has certain characteristic physical stigmata, such as a small stature with a round small head, epicanthic folds, upward and outward slanting palpebral fissures, low set oval ears, short inturning little fingers (clinodactyly), a transverse palmar crease (simian), and an enlarged deeply fissured tongue which is all in keeping with a diagnosis of Down's syndrome. (Don't ever say Mongolism which is a term not looked upon favourably and now obsolete.)

Examiner

Is there anything else that you would like to examine?

Candidate

Yes, I would like to make a formal examination of his heart for cardiac murmurs.

Examiner

What cardiac lesions would you expect in this condition?

Candidate

Down's syndrome is classically associated with an endocardial cushion defect which varies in severity between affected individuals and may contribute to a VSD, ASD or even tetralogy of Fallot. In 30% of affected individuals more than one lesion is found.

Examiner

What is the genetic abnormality in these patients?

Candidate

The majority of cases have trisomy 21, i.e. these patients have 47 chromosomes instead of 46 due to the presence of an extra chromosome 21. In some cases it is due to mosaicism or translocation of the chromosomes.

Discussion on Down's syndrome

Down's syndrome or trisomy 21 is characterized by mental

deficiency, muscular hypotonia, brachycephaly, short stature, slanted eyes, a flat nasal bridge, short broad hands with transverse palmar creases, a high arched palate, cataracts and congenital heart disease. These patients are more prone to leukaemias and on postmortem generally have a small frontal lobe. In approximately 95% of cases trisomy 21 results because of non-disjunction during meiosis; 4% are a result of translocations, and the remaining 1% occur as a result of mosaicism.

Looking at the Patient

CASE 10 SYSTEMIC LUPUS ERYTHEMATOSUS (SLE)

Examiner

Look at this woman's face, describe what you see and tell me what you think the diagnosis is.

Locally

- The 'butterfly distribution' of the erythematous skin rash over the bridge of the nose extending to both cheeks will be obvious and will alert you to the diagnosis of SLE and to look for its features.
- In this rash look for areas of scarring, telangiectasia, keratotic plugging, hypopigmentation (at the centre) and hyperpigmentation (at the edges).
- Look for alopecia.

Elsewhere

- Arthropathy of the hands with involvement of MCP and PIP joints.
- Ulnar deviation of the fingers.
- Subluxation of the PIP joints.
- Pleurisy/pleural effusions.
- Heart murmurs and pericardial rub.

Candidate

This young woman has several distinctive features which make me think of a particular diagnosis. The most striking feature is that of a butterfly-shaped erythematous rash involving her cheeks and the bridge of her nose. This rash is slightly elevated with some telangiectasia. She also has a degree of scalp alopecia. Her hands are confirmatory, in that she has periungual erythema and fusiform swelling of most of her MCP and PIP joints on both hands, suggestive of a polyarthropathy. I think that the most likely diagnosis is systemic lupus erythematosus (SLE).

Examiner

What tests would you like to perform to confirm your clinical suspicions?

Candidate

To confirm the diagnosis of SLE, I would screen for the auto-antibodies ANA, anti-dsDNA and anti-Sm. Anti-nuclear antigen (ANA) is positive in up to 95% of cases, though it is not specific for this condition. Both anti-dsDNA and anti-Sm are specific for this disease, though they are only positive in approximately 70% and 30% of cases respectively. Other auto-antibodies worth screening for include anti-Ro and anti-La, both of which are positive in ANA negative SLE, and anti-RNP which is often positive in mixed connective tissue diseases, where SLE occurs as a component. Additional tests would be to confirm disease activity and the extent of involvement of organ systems in the body.

Examiner

What additional tests did you have in mind?

Candidate

To assess disease activity the patient should have their acute phase response measured, the simplest test being that of the ESR. This is a rather crude assessment which, while not correlating with disease activity in the majority, nevertheless has a non-specific alerting role and indeed for some patients may correlate with disease activity. The CRP has no relationship to the disease and if elevated one should suspect superadded infection. The measurement of complement should be performed in all cases as low levels of C_3 and/or C_4 together with a reduced CH_{50}, are invariably associated with disease activity. (SLE is a multisystem disease and therefore every system requires assessment. Nevertheless involvement of certain systems is either more common or more easily assessed by the tests currently available.) Thus, a full blood count is required due to associated anaemia, leucopenia, lymphopenia and thrombocytopenia. The partial thromboplastin time should be measured and, if prolonged, anti-cardiolipin antibodies screened for. The presence of these may have predictive potential as to the development of certain complications such as recurrent venous and arterial thromboses and recurrent miscarriages. The respiratory system should be assessed radiologically, the renal system assessed biochemically and by examining the urine for casts.

Examiner

Do you know of any drugs that may cause a lupus-like syndrome?

Candidate

There are a range of drugs that can cause this condition. The two drugs most likely to cause this problem are: 1. procainamide, 2. hydralazine. Other drugs include: isoniazid, chlorpromazine, d-penicillamine, methyldopa, and oral contraceptives.

Examiner

Are there any unusual features of drug-induced lupus?

Candidate

Clinically, most patients with this syndrome suffer from polyarthralgias and systemic symptoms. They do not experience renal and CNS involvement. Their pattern of auto-antibodies is distinctive in that they are all ANA positive with anti-histone antibodies present in the majority (95%). Anti-dsDNA antibodies are absent.

CASE 11 SCLERODERMA (SYSTEMIC SCLEROSIS)

Examiner

Observe this woman's face and tell me what the diagnosis is.

Locally

- Classical facial appearance: thickened, taut and waxy skin with thin hairs around the lips and a pinched nose should give a high index of suspicion of the diagnosis.
- Look for telangiectasia which may be present on the face, lips, tongue.
- Demonstrate that she has a small mouth (ask her to open the mouth).

Elsewhere (with the examiner's permission)

- Examine the hands:
  - Tight, thickened skin over the fingers with disappearance of normal skin folds over the knuckles.
  - Joints may be swollen due to polyarthralgia.
  - May have ulceration at tips of fingers.
  - Look for digital vasculitis.
  - Subcutaneous calcification may be felt at tips of fingers.

Candidate

This lady's face displays evidence of sclerodermatous changes as evidenced by its smooth, wrinkle free, waxy appearance; the thin pinched nose; the small mouth limited in the extent to which it can be opened; and the facial telangiectasia. (Examine briefly the hands.) The diagnosis of scleroderma is additionally supported by the changes in her hands. The skin of the hands has a smooth, waxy appearance with limited pliability. She has developed a degree of flexion deformity of her fingers (due to the taut skin) and telangiectasia are again in evidence.

Examiner

Is there anything else that you would like to examine?

Candidate

Yes, I would like to examine this woman's respiratory system, check her blood pressure, and examine her urine.

Examiner

What tests would you request to confirm the diagnosis?

Candidate

The diagnosis can be confirmed by assessment of her auto-antibodies. Thus, I would request ANA which should be positive in at least 95% of cases. Auto-antibodies specific for this condition include anti-topoisomerase 1 (Scl-70), anti-nucleolar and anti-centromere. The presence of the latter antibody is relatively specific for the CREST syndrome. Screening for anti-RNP antibodies is useful as their presence implies an overlap syndrome (MCTD).

Examiner

What factors determine the prognosis of systemic sclerosis?

Candidate

Patients with the limited form of this disease, namely the CREST syndrome, have a relatively good prognosis. Prognosis is very dependent on the organ systems involved. Thus, renal involvement is associated with the worst prognosis, one estimate being a 30% 10-year survival while pulmonary involvement has a 50% 10-year survival. For patients with no cardiac, renal or pulmonary involvement, the 10-year survival has been estimated at 70%.

Discussion on scleroderma

Systemic sclerosis has a female:male ratio of 4:1. Any age may be affected; however, the usual age range of presentation is generally 20–50 years, with 40 years being the mean age of onset. The most characteristic features of this condition are the skin manifestations (referred to above) and the vasomotor changes (Raynaud's phenomenon), which usually result in the initial diagnosis being made. There are usually three stages in the development of the skin changes, the first phase is an oedematous one associated with stiffness, followed by the sclerotic phase and finally an atrophic phase. The sclerosis usually starts on the hands, later spreading to the forearms, face, trunk and finally the legs and feet. Dysphagia is the most common visceral symptom, occurring in over 50% of patients, while approximately a third develop radiological evidence of pulmonary fibrosis and a smaller fraction have cardiac, renal and malabsorptive complications. The major causes of death are hypertension and renal disease.

CASE 12 LUPUS PERNIO

Examiner

Look at this woman's face and tell me from what systemic condition she suffers.

Locally

- A bluish discolouration of the nose is evident and will alert you to examine for other signs of sarcoidosis.
- Look for any other skin plaques, scars or keloids.
- Examine the eyes for uveitis and choroidoretinitis.
- Examine for facial nerve palsy.

Elsewhere

- Look for erythema nodosum on the legs.
- Examine for lymphadenopathy.
- Look for bony cysts (phalanges).
- Tell the examiner that you would like permission to examine the respiratory system.

Candidate

This patient has typical swollen violaceous 4–5 cm diameter plaques on her nose and left cheek. They are indurated in nature with scattered overlying varicosities. This is the typical lesion of lupus pernio and the underlying systemic condition is most likely to be sarcoidosis.

Examiner

What other skin lesions might you expect to find in this condition?

Candidate

Skin lesions specific for sarcoidosis may be found in 10–30%

of cases and include papules distributed periorally, perinasally, on the buttocks and on the extremities. Other lesions include annular plaques, again found on the face, buttocks and extremities. Less common lesions include subcutaneous nodules and ichthyosis-like lesions. A common non-specific skin lesion is that of erythema nodosum.

Examiner

What investigations would you perform to confirm the diagnosis?

Candidate

Investigations should include:

1. Chest X-ray (hilar lymphadenopathy, infiltrates and fibrosis).
2. Serum angiotensin converting enzyme levels.
3. Biopsy of lymph node.
4. Kveim–Siltzbach test.
5. Gallium lung scan.

The diagnosis is not obtained from any one test but is a manifestation of the clinical, radiological, biochemical and histological findings.

Examiner

Does lupus pernio have any diagnostic significance apart from indicating the patient has sarcoid?

Candidate

Yes, it implies associated respiratory tract and ocular involvement.

Examiner

What are the indications for using steroids in the treatment of sarcoid?

Candidate

As such, there is no definitive curative treatment for sarcoid. Nevertheless glucocorticoids are effective in limiting the amount of tissue or organ damage, an effect which has to be counterbalanced with their long-term side effects. Thus, in certain organ systems such as the eye, the lungs, the heart and the nervous system where active inflammation is occurring, treatment with glucocorticoids is deemed appropriate.

Examiner

What is the significance of lupus pernio?

Candidate

Sarcoidosis of the upper respiratory tract is associated with an increased risk of developing lupus pernio. Early use of steroids is advocated to prevent this disfiguring complication. Kveim test is almost always positive in patients with sarcoidosis of the upper respiratory tract with lupus pernio.

Discussion on lupus pernio

Sarcoidosis is a disease of unknown aetiology, characterized by multisystem involvement. Onset is generally between 20 and 40 years of age. The disease may be self-limiting in up to 50% of patients, presenting with an acute episode with no sequelae. The remainder may be left with some permanent organ dysfunction, which in the majority tends to be mild and non-progressive. However, in 15% to 20% of cases the disease remains active or recurs intermittently. The organ systems generally affected include the skin (see above), the lungs (BHL, fibrosis), the eyes (anterior/posterior uveitis, kerato-conjunctivitis), the nervous system (central and peripheral nerve palsies, CNS lesions), the heart (heart block, cardio-myopathy), the kidneys (nephrocalcinosis) and the lymphoid tissue (lymphadenopathy, hepatosplenomegaly).

There is no diagnostic blood test, though serum ACE levels are useful, being elevated in two-thirds of patients with active disease. Unfortunately, the false positivity and negativity of the test is high. The Kveim test is now rarely used though it is diagnostic in 70–80% of patients with a high degree of specificity. It involves the intra-dermal injection of splenic sarcoid material (Kveim antigen), with a follow-up biopsy 4–6 weeks later. A positive biopsy will show non-caseating granuloma.

CASE 13 XANTHELASMA

Examiner

From what condition might this woman be at risk, and why?

Locally

- The raised, yellow plaques around the eyelid near the inner canthus will be obvious as xanthelasmata.
- Look for jaundice in the sclera and for the presence of arcus.
- Look for swelling of the eye (periorbital oedema in nephrotic syndrome).
- Ask yourself whether the facial appearance is that of myxoedema.

Elsewhere

Look for xanthomas (palms, knuckles, tendoachilles).

Candidate

The most striking feature about this woman's face is the presence of xanthelasma (raised yellow plaques) on her eyelids, arcus senilis, and xanthoma on the dorsal aspect of the knuckles of her hands. Such findings imply that she has increased circulating levels of cholesterol and thus she is at increased risk for contracting coronary artery disease.

Examiner

What type of hyperlipidaemia might this patient have?

Candidate

The most likely type of hyperlipidaemia is that of familial hypercholesterolaemia, which is an autosomal dominant disorder resulting from a mutation in the LDL receptor. Xanthelasma and tendon xanthoma (nodular, affecting the hands, elbows and knees) tend to be prominent. Affected individuals have premature and accelerated coronary artery disease.

Examiner

What other conditions are associated with xanthelasma?

Candidate

Other conditions include:

1. Familial type 3 hyperlipoproteinaemia.
2. Diabetes mellitus.
3. Hypothyroidism.
4. Nephrotic syndrome.
5. Chronic obstructive jaundice.

Examiner

What are the three main types of xanthomas?

Candidate

These are:

1. Eruptive xanthomas: these occur as firm, raised papules with pale yellow centres over the buttocks, elbows, knees and extensor aspect of the forearms. Associations include familial lipoprotein lipase deficiency, familial combined hyperlipidaemia and uncontrolled diabetes mellitus.
2. Planar or palmar xanthomas: often yellow to orange in colour, being most commonly found in the palmar and digital creases. They occur in type III hyperlipidaemia.
3. Tendon xanthomas: these occur in the extensor tendons on the hands, elbows, knees and ankles. Most are characteristic of familial hypercholesterolaemia.

- Go over Fredrickson's or the WHO classification of hyperlipidaemias.

CASE 14 HEREDITARY HAEMORRHAGIC TELANGIECTASIA (OSLER–WEBER–RENDU SYNDROME)

Examiner

Look at this man's face and tell me what you think his presenting symptom was.

Locally

- Small, flattened telangiectasic lesions on the lips, oral and nasal mucosa, tongue, and the tips of fingers and toes.
- Anaemia is present (due to bleeding lesions).
- May have clubbing (due to aneurysms/AV malformations in the lung).

Candidate

This man has multiple telangiectasia on his lips, oral mucosa, nose and hands. The most likely diagnosis is that of hereditary haemorrhagic telangiectasia, the most common presenting symptom of which is epistaxis.

Examiner

Is there anything else that you would like to examine?

Candidate

Yes, I would like to examine his respiratory system in order to assess whether or not he has any pulmonary AV malformations.

Examiner

Is this important?

Candidate

Yes, as their presence may result in such complications as pulmonary haemorrhage; they may be sufficiently large or numerous to cause shunting (right to left) with resultant hypoxia and, additionally, they may be involved in paradoxical embolic events.

Examiner

Is there any treatment for this condition?

Candidate

There is no curative therapy, though for significant visceral AV malformations, embolization may be an option. Hormone therapy in the form of oestrogens has been shown to be effective in reducing the frequency of epistaxis.

Discussion on hereditary haemorrhage telangiectasia

Hereditary haemorrhagic telangiectasia is inherited as an autosomal dominant condition. The telangiectases may first be seen in adolescence, their number increasing thereafter, peaking between the ages of 45–60 years. Visceral telangiectases and AV malformations may occur in the lungs, liver and spleen. Patients generally require continuous iron therapy to correct the tendency to iron deficiency anaemia.

CASE 15 DERMATOMYOSITIS

Examiner

This woman complains of dysphagia. Look at her face and examine her hands and tell me what the diagnosis is.

- A rash over the skin of the face, shoulders or the arms together with the history should alert you to the diagnosis of 'dermatomyositis' and you should then proceed to looking for other features of the illness.
- A 'heliotrope' with suffusion of the eyelids may be diagnostic of this disorder.
- The hands show periungual erythema and telangiectasia.

Candidate

This middle-aged woman has a characteristic facial rash, with a violaceous heliotrope erythema associated with slight puffiness plus a diffuse mild erythema affecting the sun-exposed areas of the rest of her face. Her hands show supportive changes, with periungual erythema and telangiectasia, and the presence of Gotton's papules (lichenoid papules) on the dorsum of her fingers. These findings are suggestive of dermatomyositis.

Examiner

Is there anything else that you would like to examine to confirm your clinical suspicion?

Candidate

Yes, I would like to assess the strength of her muscles to test for the pattern of a proximal myopathy, and in view of the association with malignancy I would also examine for adenopathy, breast lumps, respiratory and abdominal pathology.

Examiner

What investigations would like to perform to confirm your diagnosis?

Candidate

Laboratory investigations to confirm the diagnosis would include:

1. Serum CPK and transaminases.
2. An electromyogram (fibrillations and polyphasic discharges).
3. A muscle biopsy.
4. Barium swallow (atonic dilated oesophagus).

Additional investigations would be directed at excluding an underlying malignancy or the association with another connective tissue disease(s) in a MCTD syndrome.

Examiner

What is the relationship between dermatomyositis and neoplasia?

Candidate

The association is a paraneoplastic syndrome. It is more common in the over 60-year-olds, and may in some cases precede the diagnosis of malignancy by several years. Malignancy is rare in children and in those patients with a co-existing connective tissue disorder. The most common malignancies include those of the lung, breast, ovary and gastrointestinal tract and myeloproliferative disease.

Examiner

Assuming that there is no underlying malignancy, how would you treat this patient?

Candidate

The treatment of choice remains that of steroids usually in the form of prednisolone at 1 to 2 mg/kg/day. Improvement varies between patients though it may require anything from 1 to

4 weeks for this to occur. When there is no longer any evidence of disease activity and maximum recoverable power has been achieved, the prednisolone may be slowly tapered. A maintenance dose for several years may nevertheless be required.

Examiner

What is the prognosis of this condition?

Candidate

In those cases where there is an underlying malignancy, the prognosis is that of the malignancy. For the rest, a 5-year survival figure is estimated at 75%. Relapse may occur at any time. Most patients make a full functional recovery; however, after five years 20% may still have active disease and a further 30% may have inactive disease but with some residual weakness.

CASE 16 DYSTROPHIA MYOTONICA

Examiner

Look at this man's face and tell me what you think the diagnosis is.

Locally

- The frontal balding, wasting of face and neck muscles (especially the sternomastoids) and the bilateral ptosis are characteristic *facies* for this condition and you should not miss these.
- Look for cataracts.

Elsewhere (with the examiner's permission)

- The distal parts of the limbs may show muscle wasting.
- Check the grip of the hands on both sides and look for slow relaxation of the muscles (myotonia).

Candidate

This man has a characteristic facial appearance, with frontal balding, marked wasting of his temporalis and sterno-cleidomastoid muscles, and bilateral ptosis. This spectrum of clinical signs would make me strongly suspect a diagnosis of dystrophia myotonica.

Examiner

From what other problems do these patients suffer?

Candidate

Such patients may have a degree of mild mental impairment; they also develop posterior sub-capsular cataracts, cardiac conduction defects, hypoventilation, gastrointestinal dysmotility, and gonadal atrophy.

Examiner

Are there any laboratory tests to confirm the clinical diagnosis?

Candidate

The diagnosis is usually based on the clinical findings, the EMG pattern and to a lesser extent the presence of cataracts. In such patients the muscle enzyme levels are normal, the muscle biopsy shows non-inflammatory changes with type I fibre atrophy, which though distinctive is not diagnostic.

Examiner

Do you know of any acquired causes of myopathy?

Candidate

Yes, there are a range of conditions that can induce a myopathy. These acquired causes can be subdivided into inflammatory, endocrine and metabolic, toxic, and those associated with malignancy:

1. Inflammatory:
    a. Connective tissue diseases.
    b. Sarcoidosis.
    c. Infective, e.g. viral, protozoal and parasitic.
    d. Idiopathic polymyositis.
2. Endocrine and metabolic:
    a. Hypo-/hyper function of the thyroid, adrenal and parathyroid glands.
    b. Electrolyte abnormalities.
3. Toxic:
    a. Alcohol.
    b. Nerve gas.
4. Malignancy:
    a. Any malignancy (occur as part of paraneoplastic syndromes).

Examiner

Tell me something about facioscapulohumeral muscular dystrophy.

Candidate

This an autosomal dominant condition which, although it does not alter life expectancy, causes morbidity. The patients present with bilateral, symmetrical weakness of facial and sterno-clavicular muscles. Patients may have bilateral ptosis. The pelvic girdle and lower limb muscles may also become involved in later years. There may be loss of (or diminished) reflexes in the affected muscles with no sensory deficit.

Discussion on dystrophia myotonica

This condition is inherited in an autosomal dominant fashion, being transmitted by a mutant gene on the long arm of chromosome 19. Treatment is limited to ameliorating the complications. If the myotonia is severe, phenytoin is the treatment of choice: the other anti-myotonia agents such as quinine and procainamide may aggravate any co-existing cardiac conduction defect.

CASE 17 MYASTHENIA GRAVIS

Examiner

This young woman complains of problems with chewing her food and finishing her meals. Would you like to examine her face and tell me what the diagnosis is?

The examiner's description should make you think of conditions associated with dysphagia (e.g. bulbar problems) or a muscle fatigue problem. Therefore examine the cranial nerves in the standard fashion, previously described, looking for any evidence of lower motor neurone weakness or fatiguability. The latter is most easily elicited in testing the eye movements, with inducibility of diplopia and the development of bilateral ptosis on sustained upward gaze.

Locally

- Note the ptosis with normal sized pupils (this will give the clue to the diagnosis of myasthenia gravis).
- Examine the ocular movements (diplopia).
- Examine cranial nerves.

Candidate

This patient has very mild bilateral ptosis at rest which is accentuated on sustained upward gaze, with the development of diplopia in all quadrants on repeated testing of her eye movements. She displays a mild so-called 'myasthenic snarl' on being asked to show her teeth and, on counting serially, her speech becomes progressively slurred, nasal and of a reduced volume. There is no evidence of any cranial nerve palsies and in view of the signs elicited, the most likely diagnosis is that of myasthenia gravis.

Examiner

How would you confirm your diagnosis?

Candidate

This would be confirmed by performing a 'tensilon test'. Edrophonium hydrochloride (tensilon) is a short-acting anticholinesterase which is given as an intravenous bolus of 10 mg. In cases of myasthenia gravis, a rapid and convincing strengthening of muscle power is seen in less than a minute.

Examiner

Are there any other relevant investigations?

Candidate

a. Confirmatory investigations include:
1. Repetitive nerve stimulation.
2. Anti-acetylcholine receptor antibodies (anti-AChR).

Anti-AChR antibodies are detectable in approximately 80% of all myasthenic patients. There is little correlation between the antibody level and the severity of the disease at the time of diagnosis; however, at an individual level they may be useful for monitoring response to therapy.

b. Investigations for associated conditions:
1. Lateral CXR, CT/MRI scan of the anterior mediastinum looking for a thymoma.
2. Thyroid function tests (associated hyperthyroidism in 3–8% of cases).
3. Auto-antibody screen.

Examiner

What is the treatment of this condition?

Candidate

There are several therapeutic options; these include:

1. Oral long-acting anticholinesterases, such as pyridostigmine. Most patients benefit, though it is not a cure

and there are muscarinic side effects plus the potential of overdosage resulting in increased weakness due to desensitization of the neuromuscular end plate.

2. Immunosuppression:

   Steroids are nearly always effective in improving muscle weakness, though it tends to be a long-term therapy. Unlike most other conditions where steroid therapy is used, the initial dose tends to be quite small at 10 mg to 15 mg/day. This is then progressively increased to a maximum of 50 mg/day or 100 mg on alternate days. Improvement may continue over a period of months.

   Other drugs that are used as steroid sparing agents include azathioprine and cyclosporine. Cyclophosphamide is used for refractory cases.

   Plasmapheresis is effective in removing the pathogenic antibodies from patients *in extremis* or to improve patients' condition prior to surgery.

   Thymectomy is indicated for the removal of a thymoma. Additionally, a thymectomy in those patients with no evidence of a thymoma is indicated as it improves the myasthenia in up to 85% of patients and up to a third may obtain a drug-free remission.

CASE 18 ANKYLOSING SPONDYLITIS

Examiner

This man has noticed increasing difficulty in bending down to tie his shoe-laces. Would you care to make an assessment and tell me what you think the diagnosis is.

Locally

- After introducing yourself, clearly explain to the patient what you want him to do. Gauged from the examiner's question, the patient may be suffering from a spinal problem, a neurological problem or a muscle problem. Your decision on which it is, is dependent on your observation of the patient bending to tie his shoe-laces. At all times make sure that the patient is not inconvenienced.
- Note the characteristic posture on standing, with loss of his lumbar lordosis, buttock atrophy, mild thoracic kyphosis and a forward stooping neck.
- Confirm your suspicions by noting the marked limitation of flexion, extension and rotation of his spine, together with his limited chest wall expansion on maximal inspiration.

Elsewhere

- Look for aortic regurgitation.
- Examine lungs for apical fibrosis.
- Examine the eyes for uveitis.

Candidate

This patient has features of ankylosing spondylitis as evidence by ... (give all your physical findings).

Examiner

What tests would you do to confirm your clinical suspicions?

Candidate

There is no diagnostic lab test. I would request:

1. ESR and CRP (elevated).
2. Full blood count (a mild normochromic normocytic anaemia in an untreated patient).
3. X-ray of the sacroiliac joints, lumbar, thoracic and cervical spine. The radiological findings are characteristic, though their specificity is dependent on the stage of the disease. Radiologically there is bilateral sacroiliac joint involvement, with blurring of the cortical margins of the subchondral bone, followed by erosion and sclerosis. End-stage involvement is that of ankylosis and obliteration of the joints. Vertebral involvement starts in the lumbar region, again with osteitis, erosions and sclerosis producing a squaring of the vertebral bodies. Subsequent involvement of the annulus fibrosis leads to syndesmorphyte formation and eventual ankylosis of the spine.
6. Chest X-ray (apical fibrosis).
7. HLA typing (HLA B27).
8. Lung function tests.

Examiner

What pattern of spirometry readings would you see?

Candidate

Since the problem is a restrictive defect due to spinal ankylosis the vital capacity is reduced but the forced expiratory volume remains normal.

Examiner

What are the complications of this condition?

Candidate

The complications may be subdivided into three categories:

1. Associated extra-articular conditions:
    a. Anterior uveitis.
    b. Aortic incompetence.
    c. Amyloidosis.
2. Those related to the bony involvement:
    a. Spinal fracture with resultant cord problems.
    b. The cauda equina syndrome.
    c. Pulmonary mycetoma secondary to apical fibrosis and cavitation.
3. Those that relate to therapy:
    a. Use of NSAIDs may result in GI haemorrhage and interstitial nephritis.
    b. Previous usage of deep X-ray treatment led to increased episodes of leukaemia and post-radiation GI and renal obstructive problems.

Examiner

What is the available treatment today for these patients?

Candidate

This involves the use of regular exercise plus NSAIDs. Sulphasalazine has been shown to be a useful adjunct, in that it reduces the systemic inflammatory response as well as the symptoms of the peripheral arthritis. Surgery is also of use in providing relief and increased mobility to those patients with severe hip arthritis, marked flexion deformities of the spine and atlanto-axial subluxation.

CASE 19 TURNER'S SYNDROME

Examiner

This woman was referred to the cardiologist with a murmur. Examine her general appearance only and tell me from what condition she suffers and the most likely nature of the murmur.

- Note the short stature, webbed neck and micrognathia which should alert you to the diagnosis.
- Look for a shield chest (broad chest with widely apart nipples and poorly developed breasts).
- Examine the heart for coarctation of the aorta and pulmonary stenosis.
- Note the short fourth metacarpals.
- There is an increased carrying angle of both elbows.

Candidate

This patient has several characteristic features, such as short stature, webbing of the neck, low hair line, micrognathia, low set ears, short fourth metacarpals and mild lymphoedema of her hands which indicate a diagnosis of gonadal dysgenesis or Turner's syndrome. The most common cardiac-related abnormality is that of coarctation of the aorta; however, this patient has pulmonary stenosis.

Examiner

What other feature might you expect?

Candidate

Impaired secondary sexual characteristics, thus she would have impaired breast development with a so-called shield-like chest and widely spaced nipples.

Examiner

What single investigation would you ask for to confirm your diagnosis?

Candidate

I would ask for the cytogenetic analysis of a buccal smear; I would expect to see the karyotype 45XO or in 25% of cases 45XO/46XX. The short stature and other somatic features are thought to develop as a result of the loss of genetic material in the short arm of the X chromosome.

Discussion on Turner's syndrome

Turner's syndrome (gonadal dysgenesis) is the most common cause of primary ovarian failure. The incidence is approximately 1 in 3000 live female births. The ovaries are usually represented by streaks of fibrous tissue with no germ cells. The resultant lack of the sex hormones accounts for the absent secondary sexual characteristics.

Congenital renal abnormalities (horseshoe-shaped kidneys or double ureters) may be present in some cases. Additionally, there may be a tendency to keloid formation, hypoplastic nails, and perceptive hearing loss. If menstrual function and reproduction occur in a patient with Turner's phenotype, this must be due to mosaicism, e.g. 45XO/46XX, 45XO/47XXY.

CASE 20 LAURENCE–MOON–BIEDEL SYNDROME

Examiner

This patient attends a special school and has significantly impaired vision. What is the most likely diagnosis?

- Note that the patient is obese and short.
- Examine eyes: visual acuity; visual fields; fundi (retinitis pigmentosa); optic atrophy.
- Note that the patient is mentally subnormal from the history (you may want to perform a mental test score).
- Examine the hands and feet (polydactyly; syndactyly; scar of finger separation operation).
- Do not proceed to examine for genital hypoplasia without the examiner's permission.

Candidate

This patient is somewhat small and overweight and appears mentally deficient. He also has polydactyly and in view of the insulin chart above his bed I assume that he is also an insulin dependent diabetic. These features, together with the impaired vision, are suggestive of Laurence–Moon–Biedel syndrome.

Examiner

What are the visual problems due to?

Candidate

They are due to retinitis pigmentosa.

Examiner

How is the condition inherited?

Candidate

It is inherited in an autosomal recessive manner.

Examiner

Where is the lesion in this syndrome?

Candidate

It is thought to be in the hypothalamus.

Discussion on Laurence–Moon–Biedel syndrome

This condition is characterized by high parental consanguinity, the greatest incidence being found in Switzerland. It is characterized by dwarfism, hypogonadism, obesity, mental retardation, polydactyly and retinitis pigmentosa. The lesion is thought to be present in the hypothalamus. Diabetes mellitus may be associated. Most patients are totally blind by the age of 30 years. There is no satisfactory treatment.

CASE 21 PARKINSONISM

Examiner

This man has complained of increasing difficulty in writing. Observe his face and then examine what you regard as relevant to establish the diagnosis.

- Note that the patient is elderly and has an expressionless (mask-like) face. This should give you the clue to diagnosis.
- A pill-rolling tremor is present (movements of thumb and fingers – see Case 88)
- Ask patient to walk (short shuffling gait; absence of swinging of arms; festinant gait; hypokinesis).
- Ask patient to write (micrographia).
- Check for presence of other extrapyramidal signs such as cog-wheel rigidity (to test for it shake patient's hand and pronate the forearm).
- Test for the glabellar tap sign (on repeated tapping of the glabella the Parkinsonian patient continues blinking).

Candidate

This elderly man has a stooped posture, evident even while sitting, plus a drooling, unblinking, expressionless face. He also displays a resting, slow coarse tremor in both upper limbs with pill-rolling movements of the thumb and fingers of his right hand. There is cog-wheel rigidity in his upper limbs and he has a festinant gait.

Examiner

What is the pathology underlying Parkinson's disease?

Candidate

Parkinson's disease is due to the degeneration of the pigment-containing cells of the substantia nigra and locus coerulus with resultant deficiency of the neuro-transmitter dopamine within the caudate nucleus and putamen. Thus, it is a degenerative disease affecting the nigrostriatal dopaminergic system.

Examiner

Do you know of any other conditions which have associated parkinsonian features.

Candidate

Yes, there is a range of conditions with varying degrees of parkinsonian features; these include:

1. Arteriosclerotic parkinsonism.
2. The 'punch drunk' syndrome.
3. Striatonigral degeneration (Shy–Drager syndrome).
4. Progressive supranuclear palsy.
5. Drug-included, e.g. neuroleptics, MPTP (1-methyl-4-phenyl-1,2,3,6-tetrahydropyridine), phenothiazines.
6. Toxic, e.g. copper (Wilson's disease), manganese, carbon monoxide.
7. Postencephalitic.
8. Neoplasms.

Examiner

What is the available treatment for Parkinson's disease?

Candidate

A curative treatment does not exist. There are several different groups of drugs available which may help to alleviate the patient's symptoms.

1. Anticholinergics: the anticholinergics may be used in the treatment of rest tremor in the early stages of the disease.
2. Amantidine: this induces the release of stored dopamine and may also be useful in the initial stages.
3. Levo-dopa (helps only the dyskinesia, not tremor).

4. Bromocriptine: this is a direct dopamine receptor agonist and again plays predominantly an adjunctive role. L-dopa is the mainstay of therapy, restoring towards normal the neurotransmitter balance between dopamine and acetylcholine, improving the akinesia and postural disorders. The L-dopa is often combined with a dopa-decarboxylase inhibitor, the latter failing to cross the blood brain barrier. Such a combination limits the peripheral side effects of L-dopa, while maximizing the delivery of L-dopa to the CNS. The last group of drugs to be mentioned are the monoamine oxidase B inhibitors (e.g. selegiline). These drugs inhibit the breakdown of dopamine thus prolonging its effects. They tend to be used in combination with L-dopa.

Examiner

Does L-dopa therapy improve the tremors?

Candidate

No, the tremors may even be aggravated. L-dopa is predominantly of use in the treatment of the dyskinesia. Thus, an anticholinergic is additionally used to treat the tremor.

Examiner

What are the side effects of L-dopa therapy?

Candidate

These may be classified as short-term intermediate, and long-term side effects.

1. Short term include: nausea, vomiting, constipation, postural hypotension and cardiac dysrhythmias.
2. The intermediate group consists of mental confusion and hallucinations.
3. Long-term side effects: the so-called 'on–off' phenomenon may occur.

CASE 22 CHOREIFORM MOVEMENTS

Examiner

Look at this patient. Describe what you see and tell me what the diagnosis is likely to be.

Usually patients with either Huntington's chorea or rheumatic chorea will be shown.

- The rapid, jerky movements with no purpose (quasi-purposive) will be evident on looking at the face and distal parts of the arms and legs.
- Look at the tongue too for these movements. Ask the patient to put his tongue out (unsteady).
- If limited to one side of the body then the condition is called hemichorea.
- Ask the patient to state his name and address. Dysarthria with a slow and slurred speech is present.
- With the examiner's permission, carry out testing of the 'mental test score'. Dementia is a feature of Huntington's chorea.

Candidate

This patient displays a general restlessness, with widespread irregular, jerky, rapid movements affecting his face, trunk and limbs. This patient is suffering from a movement disorder which is best described as that of a generalized chorea. The most likely diagnosis is that of Huntington's (or Sydenham's) chorea.

Examiner

What is the mode of inheritance of Huntington's chorea?

Candidate

Autosomal dominant.

Examiner

What are the other causes of chorea?

Candidate

Apart from Huntington's and rheumatic (Sydenham's) chorea, the causes of chorea are:

1. Chorea gravidarum.
2. Senile chorea.
3. Wilson's disease (other features: cirrhosis, Kayser–Fleischer rings in cornea, haemolysis).
4. Post-encephalitis.
5. Drug-induced (e.g. phenothiazines, L-dopa).

Examiner

Tell me about Huntington's chorea.

Candidate

This is an autosomal dominant condition characterized by choreoathetoid movements and progressive dementia, usually with its onset in the late 30s. The onset of the disease is usually insidious, the full-blown clinical manifestations, in addition to those mentioned, may include seizures, dysarthria, dysphagia, postural instability, hallucinations, delusions, mania and depression. Most patients are dead within 10 to 15 years of onset.

Examiner

Can the onset occur at ages other than that which you have indicated?

Candidate

Yes, the disease may present at a younger age, although it tends then to be much more aggressive. It may even occur in childhood where it is referred to as Westphal's variant. Again this is a more severe presentation, characterized by rigidity, convulsions and cerebellar ataxia.

Examiner

Where is the lesion in chorea?

Candidate

The lesion is within the basal ganglia. There is marked atrophy of the caudate nucleus and to a lesser extent the putamen and the globus pallidus, due to neuronal atrophy. Neurochemically there is a marked decrease in the levels of γ-aminobutyric acid (GABA) and its synthesizing enzyme, glutamic acid decarboxylase.

Examiner

What treatments are available for choreiform movements?

Candidate

The dopa depletors tetrabenazine and reserpine and the dopa receptor blockers haloperidol and pimazide have been used with varying degrees of success.

Looking at the Patient

CASE 23 HEMIBALLISMUS

Examiner

Observe this patient and then tell me where the neurological lesion is.

This case is usually given to see whether you can recognize the characteristic movements.

- Note the violent, rapid, flinging limb movement from full extension into abduction or external or internal rotation.
- Get the terminology right: ballismus/ballism is bilateral but hemiballismus/hemiballism is unilateral (confined to one side of the body).
- Sometimes there are similar abnormal movements of the head.

Candidate

This man displays uncontrolled violent, rapid flinging movements of his left arm and leg. This man has hemi-ballismus, the appropriate lesion being in his right (i.e. contralateral) subthalamic nucleus.

Examiner

What lesions in particular?

Candidate

Thrombosis or embolism of the vessels supplying the sub-thalamic nuclei.

Examiner

Is there any treatment?

Candidate

Phenothiazines may be of some use in limiting the extent and frequency of these movements. Dopamine antagonists such as sulpiride and tetrabenazine may help.

What is Gilles de la Tourette's syndrome?

This is an autosomal trait, characterized by tics and behavioural problems. Tics or habit spasms are purposeless, repetitive, involuntary contractions of muscles of the face, shoulder or arm. The tics in this syndrome begin in childhood and progressively worsen. Mental functions generally remain intact. Phenothiazines may be of some use in controlling the abnormal movements.

Discussion on hemiballismus

Hemiballismus is characterized by forceful, flinging and violent movements of mainly the proximal parts of the limbs of one half of the body. The movements disappear during sleep. The most common aetiology is that of a vascular event in the contralateral subthalamic nucleus; other causes include an expanding AV malformation, trauma, tumour and multiple sclerosis. In cases of intractable involuntary movements, surgery may be indicated.

CASE 24 TITUBATION

Examiner

Observe this patient and then examine whatever system you think is appropriate.

- The vertical oscillations of the head (bobbing to and fro) will give you the diagnosis as titubation.
- Note that the oscillations are present when the patient is sitting or standing. These movements disappear if the patient is lying down.
- Go on to examine for cerebellar signs:
  - Nystagmus.
  - Intention tremor or finger–nose testing.
  - Dysdiadokonesis.
  - Ataxic gait (ask patient to walk with one foot in front of the other).
  - With the examiner's permission, ask the patient to give his address and note the scanning speech (dysarthria).
- Look for pallor of the optic disc.

Candidate

This patient has marked titubation of his head and has horizontal nystagmus ... (go on to give your findings).

Examiner

Where is the lesion which causes titubation?

Candidate

Titubation indicates disease of the cerebellum or its connections and is commonly seen in multiple sclerosis.

Examiner

What are familial tremors?

Candidate

These so-called benign essential tremors usually appear in early adult life and tend to be hereditary in origin. They are not present at rest, occurring with movement and being aggravated by emotion. If severe, beta blockers such as propranolol may be of use; alcohol also gives relief. There is no sinister underlying pathology.

Discussion on titubation

Titubation is characterized by tremors of the head or trunk at a frequency of 3–4 per second. Midline cerebellar lesions often result in such tremors which are more pronounced in the saggital plane. The tremors of titubation are faster than the head nodding found in patients with thalamic lesions.

It is possible to localize the cerebellar lesion, according to the clinical findings, as follows:

1. Truncal and upper extremity ataxia is suggestive of a lesion in the rostral cerebellum, whereas a combination of truncal and lower extremity ataxia is suggestive of a lesion in the caudal part of the cerebellum.
2. Nystagmus and intention tremors are usually present in lesions of the cerebellar hemisphere.
3. Hypotonia is a feature of a cerebellar lesion, though occasionally it may be absent in the lesions of the caudal cerebellum.
4. Dysarthria, dysmetria, and dysdiadokokinesia are usually present in lesions of the cerebellar hemisphere but absent in lesions of the rostral and caudal cerebellum.

CASE 25 PIGMENTATION OF THE MOUTH

Examiner

Examine this man's mouth and tell me what systemic disorder he has.

- Note the brown or grey discolouration/pigmentation of the mucous surface of the following:

  - Lips.
  - Buccal mucosa especially the inner aspect of the cheeks.
  - Palate.
  - Gums.
  - Side of tongue.

- Look for hyperpigmentation of the exposed parts of the body, e.g. palmar creases, hands, arms, face and neck.
- Nipples and genitalia are also hyperpigmented: this should be mentioned but not looked for without the examiner's permission.
- Note that the patient looks asthenic and, if female, there may be loss of hair, both axillary and pubic.
- Request for permission to measure the blood pressure (which is low) and to check for postural hypotension.

Candidate

This patient has brown pigmentary changes affecting the mucosal surface of his lips, and the buccal mucosa on the inner aspects of his cheeks. Examination of his palmar creases also shows hyperpigmentary changes. Such findings are suggestive of Addison's disease. To confirm my suspicions, I would check for the presence of low blood pressure and postural hypotension.

Examiner

What investigations would you perform?

Candidate

I would arrange the following investigations:

1. Random plasma cortisol level.
2. 24-hour urinary cortisols; plasma ACTH level.
3. A short synacthen test which if negative should be followed by a long synacthen test.

Examiner

What are the causes of adrenal insufficiency?

Candidate

Causes include the following:

A. Primary adrenal insufficiency (due to conditions affecting the adrenal).
   1. Autoimmune adrenal insufficiency, which is by far the most common (70%).
   2. Infection e.g. tuberculosis, fungal and viral (especially in AIDS patients).
   3. Malignant infiltration.
   4. Surgical removal.
   5. Amyloidosis.
B. Secondary adrenal insufficiency (due to conditions other than those affecting the adrenal):
   1. Hypopituitarism.
   2. Prolonged exogenous steroid therapy suppressing the pituitary–hypothalamic axis and then withdrawal.

Examiner

How do you differentiate primary adrenal insufficiency from secondary adrenal insufficiency.

Candidate

This is easily obtained by measuring the ACTH level,

which will be elevated in primary and suppressed in secondary forms of adrenal insufficiency. Clinically, there are no pigmentary changes in the secondary forms and additionally symptoms due to mineralocorticoid deficiency tend to be less marked.

Examiner

What other causes of oral pigmentation do you know of?

Candidate

Other causes include:

1. Peutz–Jegher syndrome (familial intestinal polyposis).
2. Heavy metal poisoning (arsenic, bismuth or silver intake).
3. Metastatic malignant melanoma.
4. Racial causes.

Examiner

What is your understanding of the Peutz–Jegher syndrome?

Candidate

This is an autosomal dominant condition, characterized by the presence of mucocutaneous pigmentation and multiple hamartomatous polyps in the small intestine. Unlike familial polyposis coli, it is not a pre-malignant condition.

Discussion on pigmentation of the mouth

Addison's disease is characterized by the insidious development of anorexia, weakness, weight loss, fatigue, postural hypotension, and pigmentation which affects the lips, buccal mucosa, skin folds, scars, extensor surfaces and areas of pressure or trauma. Biochemically, serum sodium, chloride and bicarbonate are all reduced, while the serum potassium is often elevated. The hyponatraemia is due to both loss of sodium in the urine (lack of aldosterone) and a shift of sodium into the intracellular compartment. Thus, the ECF is depleted of sodium and hence volume, which contributes to the hypotension. The hyperkalaemia occurs as a result of the aldosterone deficiency, the acidosis and impaired glomerular filtration.

CASE 26 LOOKING AT THE TONGUE

You may be asked to comment upon the appearance of the tongue. You should note: the size, colour, tremor, wasting, fasciculations, subfrenal ulcers, ulcers or leukoplakia on the side of the tongue, presence of candida, flattening of papilla, spasticity, etc. The following conditions may be shown.

1. Enlarged tongue (macroglossia)

Request the patient to open the mouth wide and protrude the tongue. Do not touch/handle the tongue. The tongue appears enlarged and fills the whole oral cavity. This may be seen in cases of:

a.   Amyloidosis.
b.   Acromegaly.
c.   Myxoedema.
d.   Down's syndrome.

Look for clinical features of the above conditions after requesting permission from the examiner.

2. Black hairy tongue

The filiform papillae are markedly overgrown (x4); the precise cause is unclear though it may be associated with a fungal infection. It tends to develop in individuals who are heavy smokers, or either on steroids or on broad spectrum antibiotics.

3. Geographical tongue

This condition has no significance. It is characterized by denudation of filiform papillae from areas of the dorsum of the tongue. The smooth pink mucosa contrasts sharply with normal roughened surface of the tongue and gives a maplike pattern. The pattern of denudation may vary from day to day.

4. Leukoplakia

Leukoplakia is a painless, adherent whitish patch that may develop on the buccal mucosa or tongue. It has an increased incidence in smokers, though it may also be associated with chronic trauma. It is a pre-malignant condition.

5. Carcinoma of the tongue

This occurs most commonly on the lateral borders, but occasionally it may develop on the posterior third of the dorsum or on the under surface. The tumour is usually ulcerated, with firm raised edges. In the absence of ulceration the only sign may be that of induration. Therefore a painful tongue should always be palpated.

6. Anaemia/pallor

In anaemia due to folate or vitamin B12 deficiency the tongue tends to be smooth, pale and painful, due to atrophy of the filiform papillae. There may also be angular cheilitis. In iron deficiency anaemia the tongue is often pale and smooth; however, glossitis is less marked. Patients with anaemia due to leukaemia will have swollen gingiva and bleeding gums in addition.

7. Thrush

Infection with *Candida albicans* (thrush) tends to occur as curdy white patches both on the tongue and the mucosa. The patches are easily scraped off.

8. Neurological conditions affecting tongue

Some neurological conditions affecting the tongue can be given as short cases:

a. Fasciculation of tongue and wasting (lower motor neurone disease, e.g. progressive bulbar palsy).
b. Spastic tongue with dysarthria (pseudobulbar palsy).
c. Loss of taste in the anterior two-thirds in 7th nerve palsy.

CASE 27 NEUROFIBROMATOSIS

Examiner

This man has a history of epilepsy; examine the skin of his upper limbs/thorax/other and proceed to examine him appropriately.

Locally

- The cutaneous fibromas will be prominent and will give the diagnosis away. These are commonly seen on the trunk, are discrete, movable and arranged along the line of nerves. Sometimes they are tender on pressure.
- Look for café-au-lait spots. These are coloured patches of skin pigmentation.
- Pigmentation is most commonly seen over the trunk and axillary freckling is often present.
- Look for kyphoscoliosis.

Elsewhere

- Test for deafness (acoustic neuroma).
- Examine for cerebellar signs.
- Mention the need to measure the blood pressure to the examiner (phaeochromocytoma may be associated with neurofibromatosis and there may be hypertension).

Candidate

This man has numerous macular pigmented patches on his torso resembling so-called café-au-lait patches, of which more than six are greater than 1.5 cm. He also displays axillary freckling plus numerous subcutaneous nodules, some of which are pedunculated, typical of cutaneous fibroma. Additionally, he suffers from mild kyphoscoliosis. This constellation of signs is in keeping with a diagnosis of neurofibromatosis, which would also account for his epilepsy.

Examiner

What is the commonest presentation of this condition?

Candidate

One-third present for cosmetic reasons. One-third present with symptoms of nerve compression. One-third present as an incidental finding at a routine medical examination.

Examiner

Do you know of any other conditions which have both cutaneous manifestations and epilepsy?

Candidate

Yes, there are several such conditions. These include:

1. Tuberous sclerosis where an intractable seizure problem may exist in the setting of variable mental deficiency and adenoma sebaceum (angiofibromata distributed in a butterfly distribution on the face);
2. Cerebelloretinal haemangioblastomatosis (von Hippel–Lindau syndrome);
3. Sturge–Weber disease where a capillary or cavernous haemangioma is usually limited to the cutaneous distribution of the trigeminal nerve but may be associated with a destructive venous haemangioma spreading through the subjacent leptomeninges.

Discussion on neurofibromatosis

Neurofibromatosis is an autosomal dominant condition, of which two non-allelic inheritable forms are now recognized. Type 1, carried on chromosome 7, is of the classic type, with the characteristic café-au-lait spots and tumours involving the sheaths of peripheral nerves. There may be an association with other tumours of the CNS such as optic glioma, meningioma, glioblastoma and, rarely, phaeochromocytoma. Additional associations include axillary and nipple freckling, hamartomas of the iris, mild mental retardation and stenosis of the aqueduct of Sylvius which may lead to an obstructive hydrocephalus. Type 2, carried on chromosome 22, is almost exclusively associated with acoustic neuromas which are often bilateral.

Neurofibromas originate from the Schwann cells and fibroblasts of the neurilemmal sheath of the peripheral nerve. They are of varying sizes, occur commonly over the trunk and are distributed along the course of the nerves. Some may later develop malignant changes. Sarcomatous change in the fibromas may occur. Spinal nerve root involvement can lead to cord compression. CNS fibromas may cause stenosis/compression of the Sylvian aqueduct and give rise to hydrocephalus.

CASE 28 LYMPHADENOPATHY

Examiner

Examine this patient's lymph nodes/reticuloendothelial system.

- Go over examination of all the groups of lymph nodes systematically, as follows:
- In the head and neck:

  - Pre-auricular.
  - Post-auricular.
  - Occipital.
  - Submental.
  - Submandibular.
  - Neck – Anterior triangle.
        – Posterior triangle.
  - Tonsils.
  - Supraclavicular.

- In the upper limbs:
  - Epitrochlear.
  - Axillary.

- In the abdomen:
  - Mesenteric.
  - Para-aortic.
  - Iliac.
  - Examine for spleen and liver enlargement.
- In the lower limbs/groins:
  - Inguinal.
  - Femoral.

- When enlarged lymph nodes are felt go on to ascertain the number, size, consistency, matted or not, etc.
- Make the appropriate examination, bearing in mind the range of potential causes. Clues include the presence or absence of hepatosplenomegaly, splenomegaly *per se*, the degree of adenopathy and the consistency of the enlarged lymph nodes.

Causes of generalized lymphadenopathy

1. Malignancy: acute and chronic leukaemias, lymphomas.
2. Infections:
   a. Viral (e.g. infectious mononucleosis EBV, CMV, HIV, rubella).
   b. Bacterial (e.g. mycobacterial, acute bacterial infections, brucella).
   c. Fungal (e.,g. histoplasmosis, coccidioidomycosis).
   d. Parasitic (e.g. trypanosomiasis, toxoplasmosis).
   e. Spirochaetal (e.g. secondary syphilis).
3. Connective tissue diseases: e.g. SLE, rheumatoid arthritis.
4. Lipid storage diseases.
5. Miscellaneous: e.g. sarcoidosis, amyloidosis, drug reactions, angioimmunoblastic lymphadenopathy, eosinophilic granulomatosis.

Discussion on lymphadenopathy

A definitive diagnosis in such cases is often dependent on the histology from a lymph node biopsy and/or serology, although the history and clinical examination often give a good indication of what the underlying cause is likely to be. Symmetrical lymph node enlargement with firm, non-tender glands of rubbery consistency is typical of lymphomas. In chronic infections the glands are often matted, whereas in cases of malignancy the glands tend to be hard and fixed.

CASE 29   SUPERIOR VENA CAVA SYNDROME

Examiner

This patient complains of headache. Would you care to examine him and tell me what you think the diagnosis is.

- The conjunctival suffusion and brawny oedema of the face, neck, upper arms and thorax will give you clues to the diagnosis.
- Note the prominent veins over the upper trunk with blood flowing downwards in the veins (due to development of collateral vessels).
- Examine the jugular veins which are prominent and distended.
- Look for radiotherapy markings (black outline made by the radiotherapist).

Elsewhere

- Test for hoarseness of the voice (metastatic manifestation or due to involvement of the recurrent laryngeal nerve by tumour).
- Look for finger clubbing.
- Examine the chest for signs of carcinoma, e.g. collapse, consolidation, pleural effusion.

Candidate

This patient displays the physical signs of superior vena cava obstruction. His internal and external jugular veins are prominent and elevated to the level of at least his ear lobes, with no evidence of pulsation or variation in their level with posture. There is marked conjunctival suffusion with upper limb, chest and scalp pitting oedema. The veins overlying his chest are markedly distended and the direction of flow is downwards. His fingers are heavily stained with nicotine; he is clubbed, and displays the markings of radiotherapy on the front of his chest. Clinical examination of his chest revealed a large right-sided pleural effusion. The most likely cause of this man's caval obstruction is that of bronchial carcinoma.

Examiner

What investigations would you request in order to confirm your clinical suspicions?

Candidate

I would arrange for the following tests:

1. A chest X-ray.
2. A thoracic CT scan/MRI scan to confirm SVC obstruction and to localize the origin of the cause.
3. A venogram.

To confirm the presence of a carcinoma I would arrange for:

a. Sputum cytology.
b. Pleural fluid cytology.
c. A pleural biopsy.
d. Bronchoscopy with brushings and a biopsy.

Examiner

How would you manage a patient with superior vena caval syndrome resulting from malignancy?

Candidate

The important therapeutic modalities are either radiotherapy or chemotherapy, a choice which is dependent on the susceptibility of the malignancy in question. Corticosteroids may be of use in reducing laryngeal and/or cerebral oedema.

Examiner

How does carcinoma of the lung cause this syndrome?

Candidate

Metastases in the mediastinal lymph nodes cause compression or invasion of the superior vena cava and thus interferes with the venous return.

Discussion on superior vena cava syndrome

Superior vena cava syndrome has been recognized as a clinical entity for over 200 years. Over 70% of cases are due to lung cancer, especially the right-sided tumours. Metastatic disease and lymphomas account for the majority of the remaining 30%. Occasionally tuberculous disease may be a causative factor. Onset of symptoms is generally insidious, most patients experiencing some symptoms for 2–6 weeks prior to admission. Symptoms or signs include painless swelling of the face and neck, cough, increasing dyspnoea, dizziness, headache, visual disturbance with the sensation of fullness in the ears.

CASE 30 GOITRE

Examiner

This lady has lost some weight recently and now complains of problems with swallowing. Examine what you think is relevant and tell me what you think the diagnosis is.

- The thyroid gland swelling and the history will give you the clue to focus on the neck.
- Go through a systematic examination of the thyroid (inspection, palpation, auscultation, movement with swallowing).
- Palpate both from front and from behind the patient.
- Determine the size, shape, consistency and extent of swelling and determine whether there is any retrosternal extension.
- Examine for tracheal deviation.
- Examine for tracheal compression (auscultate over the trachea).
- Examine for compression of recurrent laryngeal nerve (ask patient to speak or about a recent change in voice).
- Do not forget to listen for bruit (gland hyperactivity).
- Examine the lymph nodes of the neck (secondaries from carcinoma of the thryoid).
- Look for signs of thyrotoxicosis or hypothroidism (see Cases 4 and 5).

Candidate

This young woman has a smooth symetrically enlarged thyroid gland with an overlying bruit and no cervical lymphadenopathy. She displays signs of hyperthyroidism as evidenced by her moist sweaty palms, a resting sinus tachycardia, a fine tremor, bilateral lid retraction, lid lag and mild exophthalmos. The most likely diagnosis is that of Grave's disease.

Examiner

How would you treat this patient?

Candidate

The therapeutic options include:

1. Anti-thyroid drugs.
2. Radioactive iodine.
3. Surgery.

Initial control is best achieved with anti-thyroid drugs such as carbimazole with the adjunctive use of propranolol (to control the sympathetic overactivity), providing there are no specific contra-indications to the latter's use. If she has completed her family, radioactive-iodine is the treatment of choice; if not, then surgery in the form of a partial thyroid-ectomy or a course of carbimazole therapy for 12 to 18 months. There is a recurrence rate from both: for drugs this is approximately 50% after one year off drugs, while surgery has the potential added complication of inducing hypothyroidism. Where the goitre is particularly large and disfiguring, then surgery is the treatment of choice.

Examiner

What do you understand by the term 'endemic goitre'?

Candidate

Endemic goitre is defined as occurring when a significant proportion of the population in a given geographical area is affected. The commonest cause is that of iodine deficiency, and is therefore more common in regions far from the sea. The goitre develops secondary to excessive TSH production, which occurs as a result of the lack of an adequate negative feedback on TSH secretion by the thyroid hormones due to their impaired synthesis secondary to the iodine deficiency.

Examiner

What other causes of goitre do you know of?

Candidate

These include:

1. Dyshormonogenetic goitre: e.g. organification/coupling/ dehalogenase/iodine trap defects.
2. Drug-induced: e.g. anti-thyroid drugs, sulphonylureas, lithium.
3. Simple non-toxic goitre: (aetiology unknown, though often accounts for the majority in a non-endemic region).
4. Autoimmune thyroiditis: e.g. Hashimoto's thyroiditis.
5. Reidel's thyroiditis: (very rare; part of the group of conditions referred to as multifocal fibrosclerosis, which includes mediastinal fibrosis, retroperitoneal fibrosis, sclerosing cholangitis and orbital pseudotumour).
   Subacute thyroiditis (de Quervain's):secondary to a presumed viral thyroiditis.

CASE 31 GYNAECOMASTIA

Examiner

Examine this man's chest and tell me what you find.

- Such a statement is somewhat ambiguous unless the gynaecomastia is very obvious. In such circumstances it is best to be seen to examine both, i.e. the breasts and the respiratory system. Do not simply stop after demonstrating to your satisfaction that the patient has gynaecomastia. It could be secondary to a bronchial carcinoma.
- Make sure that the breast swellings are in fact gynaecomastia and not excessive breast fat in an obese person. Make sure the examiner sees you holding the swelling and palpating them.
- Quickly glance at the patient, asking yourself:

  - Is he tall? (Klinefelter's syndrome).
  - Is he acromegalic?
  - Is he thyrotoxic?
  - Does he have Addison's syndrome?

  If any of the above are suspected then go on to look for the features of the particular condition.
- Examine for any stigmata of liver disease (see Case 44).
- Palpate for testicular tumour (with examiner's permission).

Candidate

This middle-aged man has demonstrable bilateral gynaecomastia with other clinical signs suggestive of . . . (give the physical signs and the suspected condition; if no underlying aetiology is suspected then say so).

Examiner

What causes of gynaecomastia do you know of?

Candidate

It can occur in several conditions:

1. Physiologically in a proportion of adolescent males, with a median onset at the age of 14 years, or in old age when up to 40% of males may suffer from a mild degree of gynaecomastia.
2. Pathological causes can be divided into:
    a. Congenital, such as Klinefelter's syndrome, and androgen resistance syndromes.
    b. Acquired,e.g. conditions associated with:
        i. Increased oestrogen production such as testicular tumours, tumours producing HCG (carcinoma of the lung), liver disease, adrenal disease, and thyrotoxicosis;
        ii. Testicular failure secondary to viral orchitis, trauma, castration, etc.;
        iii. Drug-induced such as oestrogens, inhibitors of testosterone synthesis/action (e.g. ketoconazole metronidazole, spironolactone, and cimetidine) or drugs which would achieve this effect by unknown mechanisms (e.g. tricyclic antidepressants, isoniazid, busulphan and methyl-dopa).

Discussion on gynaecomastia

Enlargement of the male breast due to enlarged breast tissue is called gynaecomastia. When the enlargement is due to fatty tissue only it is termed pseudogynaecomastia. The means of differentiating the two is by mammography or ultrasonography. When the primary cause can be identified and corrected, the gynaecomastia generally resolves promptly. In those cases where it has been present for a long period, correction may not be followed by resolution due to fibrous tissue replacing the initial ductal hyperplasia. In such cases surgery is often indicated. The incidence of breast carcinoma is increased in such individuals.

PART 2

Cardiovascular System

GENERAL ADVICE

Listen to the examiner's instructions very carefully. Examine the cardiovascular system (CVS) systematically and methodically. When the examiner says something that is not clear then say so politely. For example:

Examiner   Examine this patient's heart, or Listen to this man's heart.

Candidate   I am sorry sir, but do you want me to examine the entire cardiovascular system or just restrict my examination to auscultation of the heart?

However, when the instructions are clear, go on to performing the task you have been given. For example, the examiner may say 'examine this patient's radial pulses'. Confine yourself to the radial pulses, but if there is some other examination you want to perform request the examiner's permission first, or better still present your radial pulse examination findings and then just simply say 'I would also like to examine for ...'.

Examining the whole cardiovascular system may take some time. Remember you have about five minutes only to come up with something sensible. Be quick but thorough.

Proper positioning of the patient is vital (at 45 degrees on the bed) unless the examiner specifically tells you to examine the patient sitting up (unlikely).

Make sure that the chest is well exposed.

Do not forget to examine for all the peripheral signs/clues of cardiovascular disease e.g. cyanosis, pallor, clubbing, oedema, splinter haemorrhages, Osler's nodes, Janeway spots, long marfanoid fingers, enlarged liver, ascites, dermatitis, etc. When examining the pulses make sure you look for the radial–femoral delay (or radial–carotid delay).

If you detect a raised jugular venous pulse, go through the motions of ascertaining that it is the JVP (including gently pressing on the liver) since the examiner will be bound to ask you the differences between a venous and arterial pulsation in the neck.

During auscultation, especially when a heart murmur is detected, it is expected of you:

- To time the systolic or diastolic nature of the murmur by placing the finger on the carotid artery.
- To ask the patient to 'take a deep breath in and hold it' (momentarily of course) and then to breathe out and hold the breath for a few seconds.

Similarly, during the examination of the CVS you must be seen to go through the motions of turning the patient to the left; sitting the patient up (and asking the patient to 'breathe in and hold your breath'; then 'breathe out and hold').

You must auscultate over the femorals in aortic regurgitation and in patients with atherosclerosis.

Look at the back for visible arterial pulsations (collaterals in coarctation of aorta).

Getting the patient out of bed and making him crouch down and then slowly stand up while auscultating is important in ascertaining mitral valve prolapse murmurs but should only be done with the examiner's permission; make sure the patient is fit enough to perform the procedure.

Do not forget to examine the fundi (changes of hypertension, Roth's spots, angioid streaks in Marfan's).

Auscultate the lung bases (left ventricular failure).

While 'Beri-Beri' is not common in the UK there are now Part 2 examination centres in areas of the world where it may be presented as a short case. An MRCP candidate who missed the diagnosis was told by the examiner 'young man, next time you shake the warm hands of a patient with swollen feet, think of Beri-Beri'. He was of course referring to 'high output cardiac failure'.

End your examination by telling the examiner that you want to measure the patient's blood pressure: lying down and standing. You will have to request permission to measure the upper and lower limb pressures in coarctation of the aorta.

CASE 32 MITRAL STENOSIS

Examiner

Please examine this patient's cardiovascular system.

- Malar flush may be present (but is also present with other conditions causing pulmonary hypertension).
- A small volume pulse may be present with a severe stenosis.
- Going through the examination you will note that:

  - The apex beat is tapping in quality.
  - A parasternal heave is present due to right ventricular enlargement.
  - A diastolic thrill may be present at the apex.

- The first heart sound is loud.
- Just after the second heart sound there is a sharp, short, high-pitched sound, called the 'opening snap'. It is best heard at or just inside the apex beat. With severe stenosis, the opening snap follows closely on the second sound (but with mild stenosis it is delayed).
- You will hear a murmur in the praecordial area. Note the following characteristics. The murmur is:

  - Heard in the apical area.
  - Described as rough, rumbling.
  - Mid-diastolic.
  - Best heard when the patient is asked to turn into a left lateral recumbent position. Ask the patient 'please turn over to your left side' while you auscultate.

- If the patient is in sinus rhythm, there may be a pre-systolic accentuation of the murmur.
- If the murmur is faint, getting the patient to exercise ('lie down and sit up' a few times) will make the murmur more prominent.
- Do not make the usual mistake of saying there is pre-systolic accentuation of the murmur when there is atrial fibrillation. The accentuation disappears when AF is present.
- When multiple murmurs are present (mitral regurgitation as well) try and decide which may be the dominant one

just in case you are asked. (Loud first heart sound with the presence of the opening snap favours mitral stenosis; a faint heart sound accompanied by the third heart sound is more suggestive of mitral regurgitation.)

Candidate

This middle-aged man is not cyanosed, anaemic, or clubbed, though he does display a malar flush. He is in normal sinus rhythm, at a rate of 76 beats per minute, with a small volume, non-collapsing pulse. His JVP is not elevated. On palpation his apex beat was found to be undisplaced, tapping in nature and in addition there is a right parasternal heave. Auscultation revealed a loud first heart sound associated with an opening snap. He has a mid-diastolic rumbling murmur with pre-systolic accentuation localized at his apex, which is best heard in the left lateral recumbent position. There is no evidence to support cardiac decompensation in that his lung fields are clinically clear and there is no pitting sacral or ankle oedema. These findings are in keeping with a diagnosis of mitral stenosis. His right parasternal heave is suggestive of a degree of pulmonary hypertension; however, there are no additional clinical signs to support this such as a raised JVP with prominent 'a' waves or an increased P2 with a pulmonary systolic ejection murmur.

Examiner

What three investigations could aid the diagnosis?

Candidate

1. Chest X-ray – PA and lateral views (enlarged left atrium, calcified mitral valve, upper lobe blood diversion and Kerley B lines).
2. Electrocardiogram (P-mitrale, P-pulmonale, RVH/RV strain, atrial fibrillation).
3. Echocardiogram.

How do you clinically assess the severity of the stenosis?

This may be assessed by the following three criteria:

1. The longer the diastolic murmur the more severe the lesion.
2. The shorter the interval between S2 and the opening snap the more severe the lesion.
3. Evidence of cardiac decompensation, either left or right sided, is indicative of a more severe lesion.

How is the patient affected by the development of atrial fibrillation?

Such patients have increased chances of developing heart failure and thrombo-embolic phenomena.

Discussion on mitral stenosis

Mitral stenosis is characterized by the obstruction of the flow of blood from the left atrium into the left ventricle. A positive history of rheumatic fever may be available in only 30–50% of patients; however, in greater than 90% of cases it is caused by it. Other causes include left atrial myxoma and calcification of the mitral valve annulus. Exertional dyspnoea is the most common presenting symptom; others may include palpitation, chest pain, haemoptysis and thrombo-embolic sequelae. Rarely, a patient may develop hoarseness due to compression of the left recurrent laryngeal nerve by the dilated left atrium.

CASE 33 MITRAL REGURGITATION

Examiner

Examine this patient's heart.

Ask the examiner what he really wants you to do. If he wants to restrict your examination to the praecordium only:

Locally:

- Note displaced apex beat to the left and downwards. It is strong and localized indicating left ventricular hypertrophy.
- Feel for a systolic thrill at the apex (thrills are timed as systolic or diastolic by palpating the carotid pulse at the same time as feeling the praecordial area).
- On auscultation confirm whether the patient is in sinus rhythm or not. You should hear a pansystolic murmur radiating to the left axilla.
- The first heart sound is quiet but often a third heart sound may be present due to increased return of the regurgitated blood from the left atrium.
- Look for any evidence of pulmonary hypertension (e.g. parasternal heave, loud P_2, etc.).
- Listen for associated valvular lesions, e.g. mitral stenosis.

Candidate

This patient has mitral regurgitation as evidenced by the following features: on palpation his apex beat is displaced to the 7th intercostal space, and lies 3 cm to the left of the mid-clavicular line. It is localized and strong in nature, being associated with a systolic thrill. Auscultation reveals a soft S1 with a loud pansystolic murmur which radiates to the left axilla and is associated with a third heart sound. There is no clinical evidence of pulmonary hypertension or other valvular lesions.

Examiner

What are the important causes of chronic mitral regurgitation?

These include:

1. Ischaemic heart disease.
2. Rheumatic valvular heart disease.
3. Hypertensive cardiac disease.
4. Dilated cardiomyopathy.
5. Mitral valve prolapse (congenital).

Examiner

Tell me something about mitral valve prolapse.

Candidate

An alternative name for this condition is that of Barlow's syndrome, after the physician who first described it. It is characterized by myxomatous degeneration and prolapse of one or both leaflets of the mitral valve into the left atrium during systole. The condition is more common in women and tends to be found in young adults and older age groups too (3–5% of all adults have been estimated to be affected). In most cases the lesion remains asymptomatic, the diagnosis being made on incidental clinical examination or ECHO. Symptoms, when present, commonly include palpitations, dyspnoea, chest pain, and panic attacks. The clinical findings include a mid-to-late systolic click followed by the murmur of mitral regurgitation. The prognosis is excellent, no treatment being required in the majority of cases.

Examiner

How do you differentiate a murmur of MR with that due to a ventricular septal defect or tricuspid regurgitation?

Candidate

A VSD murmur fails to radiate to the axilla; it tends to be maximal in the 4th intercostal space at the left parasternal border. TR murmur is also maximal along the parasternal border, right or left; however, it is additionally associated with giant 'V' waves in the JVP and increases in intensity on inspiration. The murmur of MR increases slightly in intensity on expiration.

Discussion on mitral regurgitation

Mitral regurgitation is characterized by regurgitation of blood from the left ventricle into the left atrium and pulmonary veins during systole. Acute mitral regurgitation can be a potentially catastrophic effect which may develop from sudden rupture of the chordae tendineae, papillary muscle or the valvular leaflet. A common cause is infective endocarditis.

In uncomplicated mitral regurgitation the apical first heart sound is faint, and is replaced by a loud blowing, pansystolic murmur which may radiate to the axilla. The apex beat, though displaced, is often strong and localized, suggestive of a degree of ventricular hypertrophy. The intensity of the heart murmur correlates poorly with the severity of the regurgitation. Common symptoms include fatiguability, exertional and nocturnal dyspnoea.

CASE 34 AORTIC STENOSIS

Examiner

This man has had several black-outs recently. Examine his cardiovascular system.

- Do a thorough examination of the cardiovascular system.
- Note the small amplitude pulse rising slowly to a delayed peak and a slow fall. There may be an extra impulse felt at the peak (then it is called an anacrotic pulse). In aortic sclerosis due to atherosclerotic hardening of the cusps of the aortic valve, the pulse is of a normal volume and character.
- Look for signs of left ventricular failure.
- Do not forget to auscultate over the carotid arteries.
- Note the displaced apex beat suggestive of left ventricular hypertrophy.
- A systolic thrill may be present.
- The second aortic sound is absent or diminished.
- Ejection mid-systolic murmur is heard, loudest at the base on expiration, usually, but not always, conducted to the right side of the neck. It may be heard all over the praecordium.

Candidate

This patient has aortic stenosis as evidenced by . . . (give your findings), or if you do not want to commit yourself just go on to give your clinical findings and say at the end that the most likely diagnosis is aortic stenosis.

Examiner

How do these patients usually present?

Candidate

Such patients commonly present in several ways:

1. The most common is that of exertional angina.

2. The second, is as exertional syncopal attacks or syncope secondary to a dysrhythmia.
3. The third is as left ventricular failure.

Examiner

What are the common causes of aortic stenosis?

Candidate

These include:

1. Rheumatic fever is the most common.
2. Congenital causes.
3. Calcification of bicuspid aortic valves.
4. Degenerative changes with calcification.

Discussion on aortic stenosis

Aortic stenosis is characterized by an obstruction to the flow of blood from the left ventricle. With significant aortic stenosis, the increasing left ventricular pressure load causes concentric hypertrophy, dilatation and dysfunction of the left ventricle. Patients may remain asymptomatic for many years. Increased oxygen requirement of the hypertrophied left ventricle and hypoperfusion of the subendocardial myocardium causes angina. Syncopal attacks typically occur on exertion. An inappropriate peripheral vasodilatation and baroreceptor response results in reduced cerebral perfusion with resultant syncope.

Angina may develop in the presence or absence of coronary heart disease. Patients with AS and cardiac failure have a poor prognosis, their life expectancy being less than two years; patients with angina and exertional syncope have a life expectancy of between 2–5 years. ECG changes may include LVH and/or LBBB. CXR may reveal cardiomegaly, pulmonary congestion and a calcified aortic valve. Cardiac catheterization is the best investigation for assessing the severity of the lesion.

CASE 35 AORTIC REGURGITATION

Examiner

Examine this patient's cardiovascular system.

- As always, start with the pulse (collapsing/water hammer pulse will give a clue to the diagnosis; pulsus bisferiens is due to combined aortic regurgitation and stenosis).
- Note the collapsing pulsation in the neck (Corrigan's sign).
- Look for signs of left ventricular failure.
- The cardinal feature of aortic regurgitation is the presence of an early diastolic murmur best heard at the left sternal edge (right sternal edge in Marfan's syndrome and syphilitic aortitis) with the patient sitting up and holding his breath at the height of expiration.
- Look for other stigmata of syphilis such as Argyll Robertson pupils.
- Auscultate over the femoral arteries (pistol shots) and test for Duroziez murmurs over the femorals (to and fro murmurs audible on slight compression of femoral artery). These are less significant signs but may be discussion points.

Candidate

This patient has aortic regurgitation as evidenced by ... (go on to give your physical signs).

Examiner

What are the causes of aortic incompetence?

Candidate

Aortic incompetence can be divided into two groups, namely acute and chronic.

1. Acute cases are much more severe with a tendency to rapid volume overload.
   a. The most common cause is infective endocarditis causing perforation or rupture of a cusp.

b. Other causes include:
   – Trauma.
   – Aortic dissection.
   The latter is more likely to occur in conditions associated with hypertension, atherosclerosis, arteritis, and Marfan's syndrome.
2. Chronic associations include:
   a. Rheumatic heart disease.
   b. Tertiary syphilis.
   c. Congenital lesions.
   d. Some of the sero-negative arthropathies such as ankylosing spondylitis and Reiter's syndrome.

Examiner

Are there any other conditions that you know of which are also associated with a 'collapsing pulse'.

Candidate

Such a pulse is a reflection of a rapid aortic run-off and has the eponymous name of 'water hammer' or Corrigan's pulse. It may also be found in patients with:

1. A large patent ductus arteriosus.
2. An aortopulmonary window.
3. A ruptured aneurysm of the aortic sinus.
4. High fever, due to the marked peripheral vasodilatation.
5. Widespread active Paget's disease.
6. Pregnancy.
7. Severe anaemia.

Discussion on aortic regurgitation

Aortic incompetence is characterized by the regurgitation of a portion of the blood back into the left ventricle; an increasing end diastolic pressure results in hypertrophy and dilatation of the left ventricle. A fall in the aortic diastolic pressure may lead to the reduction of coronary blood flow and ischaemia.

Many patients with aortic incompetence are asymptomatic for years; however, progressive regurgitation, left ventricular dilatation and eventually left ventricular failure may ensue. Exertional dyspnoea and orthopnoea are common in the late stages. Useful investigations include ECG, CXR and ECHO. ECG changes are usually those of left ventricular hypertrophy, CXR changes include cardiomegaly and if syphilis is the underlying cause calcification of the ascending aorta and/ or the aortic valve may be present. ECHO gives the most sensitive non-invasive assessment of the severity of the lesion.

CASE 36 COARCTATION OF THE AORTA

Examiner

Examine this young man's cardiovascular system.

- Go through the routine of CVS examination.
- Such a case highlights the necessity of having a comprehensive examining technique, as the answer is often given by the pulses. The ritual of checking for radial–femoral delay will pay off and its presence will arouse your suspicion as to the diagnosis.
- You will find a systolic murmur over the praecordium without cardiac enlargement.
- Look for visible/palpable arterial pulsation on the back which is best seen with the patient leaning forward. Additionally, a continuous systolic murmur may be heard in this region due to the anastomoses.
- Request permission to take blood pressure measurements in upper and lower limbs.

Candidate

The pulse is regular, at a rate of 76 beats per minute, it is of good volume and normal character. There is no radio-radial delay, however, there is marked radio-femoral delay. Palpation of the praecordium revealed a displaced heaving apex beat, located in the 6th intercostal space, 2 cm to the left of the mid-clavicular line. Auscultation revealed that the first and second heart sounds were present with an increase in intensity of the aortic component of the second sound. A mid to late ejection systolic murmur is audible throughout the praecordium, being maximal over the back. As a result of these clinical findings I think that this man has coarctation of the aorta.

Examiner

What investigations would you request?

Candidate

This patient requires:

1. Electrocardiogram.
2. Chest X-ray.
3. Echocardiogram.
4. Aortogram to define the blockage, pressures, etc.

The CXR may in itself be diagnostic due to the presence of characteristic features such as:

1. Rib notching.
2. Dilated descending aorta.
3. A figure of three sign due to indentation of the aorta at the site of coarctation with pre- and post-stenotic dilatation.

Examiner

What other causes of rib notching do you know of?

Candidate

1. Neurofibromatosis.
2. Inferior vena cava obstruction.

Discussion on coarctation of the aorta

The possibility of coarctation should always be considered in all children and young adults with hypertension. The majority of unoperated patients are dead before the age of 45 years. The usual causes of death are bacterial endocarditis, ruptured cerebral aneurysm or a dissecting aneurysm.

CASE 37 ATRIAL SEPTAL DEFECT (ASD)

Examiner

Examine the cardiovascular system.

- Signs of heart failure or infective endocarditis may be present (unlikely since the patient will be on treatment).
- The radial pulse will reveal a large volume pulse.
- Note the apex beat is not usually displaced but in some cases there may be right parasternal heave due to right ventricular enlargement.
- The diagnosis is usually obvious on auscultation: a mid-systolic murmur, left of the sternum, maximal in the 3rd intercostal space, with wide splitting of the second heart sound which is relatively fixed in relation to respiration.
- When ASD is suspected, go on to carefully listen for a murmur of mitral stenosis which, if present with ASD, is called Lutembacher's syndrome.

Candidate

This patient has clinical features of an atrial septal defect. The apex beat is undisplaced. He has a parasternal heave with a loud first heart sound, with wide fixed splitting of the second heart sound. A soft ejection systolic murmur is heard over the 2nd and 3rd intercostal spaces just to the left of the sterum and he has a soft mid-diastolic murmur which is enhanced by inspiration, maximal just to the left of the sternum, again in the 4th intercostal space. These findings are in keeping with an ASD, associated with a degree of pulmonary hypertension and relative tricuspid stenosis.

Examiner

What investigations would you ask for and why?

Candidate

1. Electrocardiogram.

2. Chest X-ray which may show cardiomegaly with pulmonary plethora (hilar dance).
3. Echocardiogram which may show the defect.
4. Cardiac catheterization.

Examiner

What would you expect to find on his ECG?

Candidate

In an ASD of the ostium secundum type, I would expect partial right bundle branch block, whereas in the ostium primum type I would expect left bundle branch block.

Examiner

What do you understand by the term Eisenmenger's syndrome?

Candidate

Eisenmenger's syndrome is the name used to describe the presence of a reversed left to right shunt associated with pulmonary hypertension. By definition it is present from birth. An acquired Eisenmenger reaction may occur in those individuals with an ASD, VSD or patent ductus arteriosus, where reversal of a left to right shunt develops secondary to the development of pulmonary hypertension. Such patients are often severely cyanosed and markedly clubbed.

Discussion on atrial septal defect

Atrial septal defects are almost always congenital in origin. The two main types are the ostium primum and ostium secundum. The former results from a failure of fusion of the septum primum with the endocardial cushion, and is commonly associated with other atrioventricular valvular defects. Ostium secundum is the most common form of congenital heart disease in adults. Most patients remain asymptomatic for many years; with small defects (less than 2 cms) patients may live into their seventh or eighth decades. With larger lesions symptoms often appear with the development of pulmonary hypertension and understandably include progressive dyspnoea and fatigue. Surgery is the treatment of choice and is indicated for all patients with significant shunts (pulmonary:systemic flow ratio of greater than 1.5). Surgical closure of an ASD at a young age (3–4 years) is usually associated with good results.

CASE 38 VENTRICULAR SEPTAL DEFECT

Examiner

Examine this patient's cardiovascular system or listen to his heart.

- Central cyanosis may be present (seen in VSD with reversed shunts – Eisenmenger's syndrome).
- There may be signs of cardiac failure or infective endocarditis.
- Note that apex beat is not displaced.
- A systolic thrill maximal in the 4th intercostal space to the left of the sternum will be present.
- Note the pansystolic murmur heard best in the 3rd or 4th left intercostal space radiating over the praecordium.
- A third heart sound is often present due to rapid filling of the left ventricle.
- Once you have a suspicion of VSD, listen for the presence of any functional pulmonary systolic or mitral diastolic murmurs which may be detected in patients with larger septal defects where the output of the right ventricle may be even double that of the left ventricle into the aorta.

Candidate

This patient has a ventricular septal defect as evidenced by ... (give your clinical findings).

Examiner

What are the indications and contra-indications for surgery?

Candidate

Indications include:

a. Right ventricular systolic pressure that exceeds 50 mmHg.
b. Pulmonary to systemic flow ratio in excess of 1.5:1 or a pulmonary to systemic vascular resistance ratio of more than 1:5.

A specific contraindication would be:

a. The presence of an acquired Eisenmenger's syndrome.

What is a Maladie de Roger?

This is a term used to describe a small VSD which is asymptomatic, has no functional sequelae and thus produces no changes on ECG or chest X-ray. Small VSDs give loud murmurs whereas larger shunts often have quieter murmurs.

Discussion on ventricular septal defect

A ventricular septal defect (VSD) is characterized by a communication between the two ventricles. The shunt is usually left to right because of the pressure differences. In >50% of cases the smaller defects may close spontaneously during the first year of life. The CXR is usually normal in patients with small to medium defects. In those with larger defects, cardiomegaly and other features of cardiac failure may be present. In such patients the ECG may show left ventricular or biventricular hypertrophy and with the development of moderate to severe pulmonary hypertension right axis deviation is common.

Other cardiac cases not discussed but which the candidate should read around and learn to recognize are:

1. Replaced artificial valves: patients who have had thoracic surgery (operation scars present) and have had their valves replaced. Read up the different types of valves (tissue versus mechanical) and familiarize yourself with the chest X-ray pictures of patients with these valves.
2. Dextrocardia (may even be part of the Kartagener's syndrome).

PART 3

Respiratory System

GENERAL ADVICE

When asked to examine the respiratory sytem you must methodically and systematically go through the ritual. You can have the patient reclined at 45 degrees on the bed or sitting up in a chair.

Start with peripheral signs of respiratory disease first and then examine the chest. When the examiner says 'listen to this patient's chest' or 'examine this patient's chest' you can go on to following the instructions and then tell the examiner that you would also like to look for peripheral signs. If you are not sure about what he/she wants you to do, do not be afraid to ask for clarification politely.

Peripheral signs should be looked for and include the following:

- Clubbing.
- Rheumatoid hands (pleural effusion or nodules).
- Wasting of the first dorsal interosseous muscles.
- Nicotine staining of fingers.
- Signs of carbon dioxide retention if indicated (warm, moist palms, hand tremors/flap, tachycardia/bounding pulse, retinal vein distension, and papilloedema).
- Examine pulse for pulsus paradoxus.
- Look on the forearm for evidence of a Kveim test (scar) or a Mantoux test.

– Look at the arm, or forearm for evidence of a BCG scar.
– Peripheral oedema (right-sided heart failure).
– Examine for lymph nodes in the axillae and neck.
– Kyphoscoliosis.
– Look at the face for butterfly rash of SLE (pleural effusions).

In addition, you should be aware of the following:

- Look for central cyanosis.
- Examine the JVP.
- Count the resting respiratory rate while examining for pulsus paradoxus.
- Look for evidence of radiotherapy markings or surgical scars or a recent pleural tap or biopsy.
- Palpate the trachea to ascertain its position or its deviation.
- Check position of apex beat.
- Inspect for chest wall movements and flattening of chest wall (collapse).
- Palpate for chest wall movements and vocal and tactile fremitus.
- Go on to percuss and auscultate (anteriorly and posteriorly).
- There may be a sputum pot (look inside it).

E 39 COLLAPSE OF THE LUNG

Examiner

Examine this man's respiratory system and give me a differential diagnosis.

- Peripheral signs may reveal signs of a possible carcinoma (nicotine staining, clubbing, etc.).
- Respiratory rate may be increased (tachypnoea).
- Note the central cyanosis (look at the tongue and buccal mucosa).
- Diminished chest movement with flattening of the chest wall on the side of the collapse.
- Shift in trachea and apex beat of the heart towards the side of the chest flattening gives the clue to diagnosis. Usually the shift of the trachea is seen if the upper lobe of the lung is collapsed, whereas if the lower lobe is collapsed it is the apex beat that is shifted towards the side of the collapse.
- Percussion note is impaired over the site of collapse.
- Breath sounds are impaired over the site of collapse.
- Bronchial breathing and crackles may be present if associated with consolidation.

Candidate

This middle-aged man is in mild respiratory distress at rest with a tachypnoea of 22 per minute. His hands show marked nicotine staining of his fingers; he is clubbed and centrally cyanosed. There is no evidence of asterixis, pallor or splinter haemorrhages. Inspection of his chest revealed a diminished chest wall movement affecting the lower right third. His trachea is slightly deviated to the right and his apex beat lies within normal limits. Palpation indicates a marked reduction in tactile fremitus also affecting the right lower third of his chest. Percussion is dull in this area though not of a stony dull nature; vocal fremitus is absent and auscultation also reveals absence of breath sounds in this area. The most likely diagnosis, compatible with these physical signs, is that of a right lower lobe collapse. An alternative might be that of a basal effusion

with underlying collapse; however, the lack of stony dullness
and the failure to detect any whispering pectoriloquy at the
upper limit of the area of dullness are against such a conclusion.
The last possibility is that of consolidation with occlusion of
the right lower main bronchus; however, this fails to explain
the finding of the tracheal deviation.

Examiner

What is the most likely cause of this man's physical signs?

Candidate

In view of the nicotine staining of the fingers and the finger
clubbing, the most likely diagnosis is that of an occluding
bronchial carcinoma affecting his right lower lobe bronchus.

Examiner

What investigations would you like to perform?

Candidate

1. Chest X-ray (PA and lateral).
2. Blood gases.
3. To establish the diagnosis, he requires sputum cytology,
   a bronchoscopy with brushings and biopsy if possible.
4. The extent of spread will require a full biochemical profile
   for assessment of liver function, bony involvement and
   paraneoplastic phenomena.
5. To assess local involvement, a thoracic CT scan, and for
   more distant spread an abdominal ultrasound scan and
   a bone scan should be performed.

Examiner

What type of paraneoplastic phenomena did you have in
mind?

Candidate

There are several paraneoplastic syndromes that can occur with bronchial carcinoma.

1. The most common group is that associated with endocrine abnormalities, for example:
    a. PTH-related peptide production by squamous cell carcinoma.
    b. The syndrome of inappropriate ADH production by small cell carcinoma.
2. Non-endocrine associations include:
    a. Hypertrophic pulmonary osteopathy usually associated with adenocarcinomas.
    b. Neurologic–myopathic syndromes including the Eaton–Lambert syndrome.
    c. Peripheral neuropathies.
    d. Subacute cerebellar degeneration.
    e. Polymyositis.
    f. A significant proportion, 1–8% may suffer from migratory venous thrombophlebitis.
    g. Non-bacterial thrombotic endocarditis.
    h. DIC.
    i. Cutaneous manifestations may include dermatomyositis and acanthosis nigricans.
    j. Renal manifestations may include the nephrotic syndrome or glomerulonephritis.

CASE 40 CONSOLIDATION OF THE LUNG

Examiner

Examine this patient's respiratory system and tell me what your clinical findings are.

- Go through the routine of examination of the respiratory system.
- Look for central and peripheral cyanosis.
- Tachycardia and clubbing may be present.
- On inspection:
  - Movement of chest wall is reduced on the affected side.
  - Trachea is central and apex beat is not shifted.
- On palpation vocal fremitus is increased and chest expansion is reduced on the affected side.
- The percussion note is impaired on the affected side (dullness).
- Carefully listen on auscultation for:
  - Bronchial breathing.
  - Fine or coarse crackles.
  - Pleural rub.
  - Whispering pectoriloquy.
  - Increase in vocal resonance.

Candidate

This unwell man displays respiratory distress at rest, with a tachypnoea of 26 per minute, fever, a tachycardia of 108 per minute and evidence of central cyanosis. His trachea is central, he has reduced expansion of this chest on the left with an area of increased tactile fremitus affecting the lower half of his left chest posteriorly. Percussion reveals this area to be dull in nature: auscultation demonstrates increased breath sounds, whispering pectoriloquy, increased vocal fremitus with coarse crepitations that alter with coughing. These clinical signs are in keeping with a diagnosis of left lower lobe consolidation. In view of this man's high temperature, the cause is most likely to be infective in nature.

What are the causes of consolidation?

The causes of consolidation can be conveniently divided into three groups, namely:

1. Infection.
2. Infarction.
3. Malignancy.

What do you understand by the term nosocomial infection?

This is an infection that is acquired by the patient during his or her hospital stay. An average figure of 5% of patients admitted to general hospitals develop a nosocomial infection. Such infections are often caused by virulent organisms; gram positive bacilli are often the most common causative organism, closely followed by gram negative bacilli. Organisms involved include *Staphylococcus aureus*, in particular the MRSA strain, *Streptococcus D*, enterobacter, *Pseudomonas* and *Serratia* although this is an ever-increasing list. A high incidence of these infections are seen in intensive care patients, burn unit patients and in dialysis patients. Certain infections may be acquired within hospitals by individuals who are not necessarily immunocompromised. Such infections may almost be as great a risk to the care giver as to the patient and include the *Hepatitis Viridiae* B and C plus the HIV virus. With the increasing number of immunocompromised patients, either from illness or treatment, an increasing number of opportunistic infections is being caused by organisms of low virulence. Thus, bacteria of low virulence such as *Staphylococcus epidermidis*, diphtheroids and fungi such as *Candida*, and *Aspergillus* are of increasing importance.

CASE 41 PLEURAL EFFUSION

Examiner

Examine this man's chest please.

This is a very common respiratory short case. Again examine carefully in a systematic fashion.

Locally

- Note diminished chest movements on the side of the effusion.
- Trachea and apex beat are shifted to the side opposite the effusion.
- Vocal fremitus is impaired or absent.
- There is stony dullness over the effusion.
- Note the absent or reduced intensity of breath sounds over the effusion.
- Vocal resonance is absent.
- Bronchial breathing may be present over the upper limit of the effusion.

Elsewhere

- Request examiner's permission to look for signs of possible causes of effusion (e.g. rheumatoid arthritis, SLE, yellow nails).

Candidate

This middle-aged man has mild respiratory distress at rest with a respiratory rate of 20 per minute. He is centrally cyanosed and clubbed; there is no evidence of pallor or carbon dioxide retention. His trachea is slightly deviated to the right, he has reduced chest wall expansion on the left as is tactile fremitus. Percussion reveals a stony dullness affecting the entire left side of his chest with markedly reduced breath sounds and vocal fremitus also on the left. These clinical signs are in keeping with a large left-sided pleural effusion.

(The clinical signs of a pleural effusion are straightforward and easily discerned; what one must be alert to is the underlying aetiology. Thus, while completing the ritual of examination you should give some thought to this question.)

Examiner

What do you think the possible causes are?

Candidate

In view of his age, the unilateral nature of the effusion and his finger clubbing, the most likely diagnosis is that of malignancy, probably a primary which could either be of pleural or parenchymal origin.

Examiner

What other causes of pleural effusion do you know of?

Candidate

Other causes include:

1. Infections (e.g. mycobacteria, pneumonia).
2. Heart failure.
3. Hypoalbuminaemic states (e.g. nephrotic syndrome).
4. Connective tissue disease (e.g. rheumatoid arthritis, SLE).
5. Pulmonary infarction secondary to large pulmonary emboli.
6. Pancreatitis.
7. Lymphatic obstruction.
8. Meig's syndrome.

Examiner

What investigations would you perform?

Candidate

1. Chest X-ray to confirm the clinical suspicion and to exclude any clues from his 'unaffected' lung.
2. Sputum should be sent for cytology and AFB staining, if available.
3. The pleural fluid should be tapped and a pleural biopsy performed, the former sent for biochemistry, cytology and AFB and the latter for histochemical analysis.
4. Bronchoscopy should be performed with the appropriate brushings and a biopsy if a lesion is visible.
5. He additionally requires:

   – Full biochemical profile.
   – Abdominal ultrasound scan.
   – Thoracic CT scan.
   – Depending on the results, a bone scan.

Examiner

Define a transudate.

Candidate

A fluid is referred to as a transudate as opposed to an exudate if its protein content is less than 2 g/litre. A pleural exudate is a more common finding, being associated with infection, malignancy, infarction and connective tissue diseases of the lung. A transudate is found when the pleural effusion is due to cardiac failure, hypoalbuminaemia, Meig's syndrome (ovarian fibroma), ascites and right-sided pleural effusion, and the yellow nail syndrome.

Examiner

Apart from the protein content of the fluid are there any other constituents that are useful clinical indicators?

Candidate

1. The pH of the fluid may be minimally useful as an acidic pH tends to be associated with conditions such as malignancy, empyema, RA, SLE and tuberculosis.
2. The glucose level is worth checking as it is typically reduced in RA, SLE and tuberculosis.
3. An amylase value of 200 units/dl is often indicative of pancreatitis or occasionally malignancy.
4. If the initial pleural tap was found to be blood stained, this suggests malignancy, infarction or trauma as the causative aetiology.
5. Chylous fluid suggests malignancy or trauma to the thoracic duct.

CASE 42 FIBROSING ALVEOLITIS

Examiner

Examine this man's respiratory system.

When examining the peripheral signs you will note clubbing. This should alert you to one of four common respiratory causes of clubbing (bronchial carcinoma, bronchiectasis, fibrosing alveolitis and lung abscess). Nicotine staining may indicate bronchial carcinoma. Basal crackles means bronchiectasis (coarse) or fibrosing alveolitis (fine).

Candidate

This man is tachypnoeic and distressed at rest, he is clubbed and markedly cyanosed centrally. He has a resting regular tachycardia of 110 beats per minute, his JVP is elevated to his earlobes and it displays prominent 'a' waves. He has pitting sacral and ankle oedema to the level of his knees. Examination of his chest revealed a central trachea with a reduced crico–sternal distance; his chest wall expansion is symmetrically reduced and percussion revealed dullness at both bases. Auscultation revealed showers of medium to coarse inspiratory crepitations affecting the lower two-thirds of his lung fields bilaterally; these crepitations failed to alter with coughing. This man displays the signs of cor-pulmonale secondary to a fibrosing condition of his lungs.

Examiner

What investigations would you do?

Candidate

To establish the severity of the condition, he requires:

1. A chest X-ray.
2. An ECG.
3. A FBC.

4. Pulmonary function tests.
5. Arterial blood gases whilst breathing air and oxygen.

From a diagnostic point of view he requires the following investigations:

6. A bronchoscopy with lavage and biopsy.
7. A lung gallium scan.
8. A CT of his thorax.
9. Other tests include: an ESR, serum auto-antibodies, SACE level, serum precipitins and immunoglobulin levels.

Examiner

Are there any questions that you would like to ask the patient which might help with the diagnostic process?

Candidate

Yes, an occupational and a pet history would be of use in assessing whether this clinical picture was a manifestation of one of the many pneumoconioses.

Examiner

Are there any drugs that can cause interstitial lung disease?

Candidate

Yes, many such drugs exist. These include:

a. Cardiovascular drugs, e.g. procainamide and hydralazine;
b. CNS drugs, e.g. amitriptyline, phenytoin and carba-mazepine;
c. Antibiotics, e.g. nitrofurantoin and isoniazid;
d. Cytotoxics, e.g. busulphan, methotrexate, and bleomycin; and a miscellaneous group which includes allopurinol, penicillamine and phenylbutazone.

Discussion on fibrosing alveolitis

Idiopathic diffuse interstitial fibrosis or fibrosing alveolitis is a condition characterized by dyspnoea, dry cough, clubbing, crepitations/crackles over the lower portions of the lungs. Some patients with rheumatoid arthritis develop similar fibrosis over the bases of the lungs. In ankylosing spondylitis the fibrosis is seen in the upper parts of the lungs. Other collagen disorders that cause interstitial pulmonary fibrosis include scleroderma and dermatomyositis.

CASE 42 KYPHOSCOLIOSIS

Examiner

Look at this man's thorax and tell me what condition he might be suffering from.

This is undoubtedly a quickie; however, you should be clear about the associated conditions and potential sequelae.

- The kyphosis (forward bending of the spine) and scoliosis (lateral bending) will be obvious.
- Note whether the kyphoscoliosis is mainly in the thoracic region or thoracolumbar region.
- Ascertain whether the curvature is to the right or left, and if there are any fused vertebrae, spina bifida or absent ribs.
- Look for hump or gibbus formation due to rotation of the spine with the prominence of the posterior angles of the ribs.
- In view of the associations look for any evidence of a Marfanoid habitus, or evidence of neurofibromatosis.
- Assess any cardiopulmonary problems as a result of the kyphoscoliosis, such as evidence of right-sided failure.

Candidate

This patient has kyphoscoliosis of the thoracolumbar spine with no evidence of gibbus formation. He has no clinical features of associated conditions such as Marfan's syndrome or neurofibromatosis.

Examiner

What two investigations would you request?

Candidate

1. X-ray of the chest and thoracolumbar spine.
2. Lung function tests.

Examiner

Name some neurogenic associations of kyphoscoliosis.

Candidate

1. Poliomyelitis.
2. Syringomyelia.
3. Freidreich's ataxia.
4. Neurofibromatosis.

PART 4

Abdomen

GENERAL ADVICE

Make sure the patient is lying flat and is comfortable. The abdomen should be fully exposed (get the cover sheet rolled up to just below the groin and cover the genitalia. Pull the patient's shirt/gown to just below the nipples).

Go systematically through the inspection, palpation, percussion, auscultation routine. Don't forget to examine for ascites (fluid thrill and shifting dullness).

Do not forget to ask the patient if there is any painful area before touching him/her. Leave examination of that area until the end and do so gently.

Check for muscle guarding and rebound tenderness in tender areas.

Do not perform a rectal examination but instead tell the examiner that you would have liked to do it.

Looking for jaundice and supraclavicular nodes is considered an essential part of the abdominal examination.

Sometimes the examiner's instructions may not be clear especially when the examiner wants you to restrict your examination solely to the abdomen while you feel that looking for relevant extra-abdominal signs would be useful. When in doubt request the examiner's permission to do so or simply say 'I have completed my examination of the abdomen but I would also like to examine the patient for other signs of liver cirrhosis such as palmar erythema, Dupuytren's, etc.'.

Examination of the scrotum for undescended testes should be done with the examiner's permission.

CASE 44 HEPATOMEGALY

Examiner

Examine this man's abdomen and tell me what you find.

Locally

- Palpation will reveal a mass in the right hypochondrium.
- Ascertain the extent of enlargement preferably in centimetres below the costal margin. Always percuss to define the upper border of the liver too (normally dull up to the 4th intercostal space).
- Make sure you have noted the following liver characteristics:
  - Liver edge: regular or irregular.
  - Liver surface: smooth or nodular.
  - Consistency: firm or hard.
  - Tenderness: present or not.
- Auscultate over the liver for bruits or rub.
- Check for splenomegaly.
- Check for ascites and caput medusae.

Elsewhere

Look for signs of liver disease:
- Check for supraclavicular nodes.
- Look for spider naevi (upper limbs, face and thorax = drainage of the superior vena cava).
- Examine nails for leuconychia.
- Examine for Dupuytren's contractures.
- Inspect for raised jugular venous pulse.
- Look for jaundice.
- Look and palpate for gynaecomastia.
- Check for testicular atrophy.
- Examine for pedal oedema.
- Look for absence of secondary sexual hair.

Candidate

(Examination should be systematic and thorough.) This plethoric, middle-aged man is jaundiced. Examination of his hands revealed leuconychia and bilateral Dupuytren's contractures, with numerous spider naevi. Palpation revealed a soft abdomen, which is non-distended and non-tender in nature. He has an enlarged, smooth, non-tender liver which extends 10 cm below the costal margin and superiorly extends to the 3rd intercostal space. There is no bruit audible over the liver. Other features of note include bilateral gynaecomastia (go on to give all your physical findings).

Examiner

What do you think are possible causes of this patient's liver condition?

Candidate

There are several possible causes:

1. Chronic active hepatitis.
2. Acute or chronic alcoholic hepatitis.
3. Infective hepatitis.
4. Infiltrative conditions such as myeloproliferative conditions, sarcoidosis, amyloidosis, haemochromatosis (lacks the classical skin bronzing) and possibly lymphoma.
5. Others include hepatocellular carcinoma, Wilson's disease, metastatic disease (hard consistency), primary biliary cirrhosis (predominates in women), hepatic vein thrombosis (expect ascites and splenomegaly) and right heart failure from whatever cause (elevated JVP, a pulsatile liver, ascites).

Examiner

What investigations would you organize?

Candidate

1. Liver function tests.
2. Liver scan (USS, CT).

3. Infective hepatitis screen.
4. Alphafetoprotein levels.
5. Liver biopsy (clotting screen first).

Below are a list of investigations one should keep in mind when discussing a liver case:

1. Biochemical investigations:
   a. Liver function tests
   b. Alphafetoprotein level.
   c. Serum iron and ferritin levels.
   d. Serum ceruloplasmin levels and urinary copper levels, serum blood glucose.
2. Haematology.
   a. An ESR and a FBC plus film.
   b. Clotting screen.
3. Serological tests include:
   a. Hepatic viral screen inclusive of hepatitis A, B and C, CMV, EBV, toxoplasma.
   b. An auto-antibody screen for ANA, dsDNA, RF, anti-mitochondrial antibody.
   c. SACE level.
   d. Anti-phospholipid antibodies.
4. Radiological investigations include:
   a. An abdominal ultrasound followed if necessary by an abdominal CT scan.
   b. If there is any suggestion of hepatic vein thrombosis, venography of the hepatic veins should be performed.

CASE 45 SPLENOMEGALY

Examiner

This young woman has had a recent sore throat and has complained of excessively heavy periods for the past couple of months. Would you kindly examine her abdomen and tell me what you find.

Locally

- Systematic abdominal examination will reveal a mass in the left hypochondrium. Make sure you start palpating from the right iliac fossa towards the left hypochondrium since a large spleen may be easily missed.
- Make sure you go through the motions of distinguishing this from a left kidney (ballotment, getting above the mass, etc.).
- Measure the enlargement in centimetres.
- Check for hepatomegaly.
- Exclude presence of ascites.

Elsewhere

- Examine for lymphadenopathy.
- Check for anaemia and jaundice.
- Examine the throat and gums (bleeds).
- Plethoric facies (polycythaemia rubra vera).
- Sternal tenderness (leukaemia).
- Splinter haemorrhages (SBE).
- Rheumatoid hands (Felty's syndrome).

Candidate

This undistressed young woman displays no stigmata of chronic liver disease and though not jaundiced she is pale . . . (go on to present your findings).

What features make you think that you have been feeling a spleen?

The features of an enlarged spleen include:

a. A palpable splenic notch.
b. Inability to get above it.
c. Dullness to percussion from the 9th rib in the left mid-axillary line, extending inferomedially in line with the predicted path that an enlarged spleen would occupy.
d. Moves with respiration.
e. Is not bimanually palpable.

What do you think the most likely diagnosis is?

In view of the sex and age of the patient (say, early 20s), the finding of splenomegaly and purpura in the setting of an insidious onset is suggestive of a haematological aetiology; the possibilities include idiopathic thrombocytopenic purpura, possibly an acute leukaemia such as acute myelogenous leukaemia and less likely infectious mononucleosis.

What investigations would you request?

The patient requires:

1. An urgent FBC plus blood film; subsequent investigations are dependent on this result. If there is selective

thrombocytopenia or numerous blasts the patient requires an urgent bone marrow and trephine examination. In the case of isolated thrombocytopenia investigations should be directed towards determining the aetiology. Investigations should include a viral screen, anti-platelet antibodies screened for plus those auto-antibodies associated with connective tissue diseases. Vitamin B12 and folate levels should also be checked and if the setting was more acute, FDPs sought and a complete infective and gynaecological screen performed. Historically any potentially marrow toxic drugs should be excluded.

Common conditions associated with splenomegaly

You should be in a position to be able to discuss a few common conditions for mild, moderate and massive splenomegaly.

Mild enlargement

1. Infective:
   a. Viral hepatitis.
   b. Infectious mononucleosis.
   c. Septicaemia.
   d. Typhoid fever.
   e. Brucellosis.
   f. Miliary TB.
2. Non-infective.
   a. Sarcoidosis.
   b. SLE.
   c. Felty's syndrome.

Moderate enlargement

1. Malignant.
   a. Chronic lymphatic leukaemia.
   b. Malignant lymphoma.
   c. Acute leukaemia.
2. Haematologic.
   a. Anaemia (aplastic, pernicious, haemolytic).
   b. ITP.

3. Infective.
   a. Bacterial endocarditis.
   b. Hydatid.
   c. Malaria.
4. Other.
   a. Sarcoidosis.
   b. Amyloidosis.
   c. Biliary cirrhosis.
   d. Portal hypertension (progresses to massive).

Massive enlargement

Five common causes are:
a. Chronic myeloid leukaemia.
b. Myelofibrosis.
c. Polycythaemia rubra vera.
d. Tropical splenomegaly syndrome (*P. malariae*).
e. Kala-Azar (visceral leishmaniasis).

Discussion on splenomegaly

Splenomegaly is a common short case in the MRCP exam, mostly given to determine whether you can pick it up and distinguish it from a kidney and that you know the common causes of splenomegaly (see Case 47). Apart from the features already discussed, the candidate must turn the patient to the right so that the splenic notch can easily be palpable in cases where there is only marginal enlargement of the spleen.

CASE 46 HEPATOSPLENOMEGALY

Examiner

Could you examine this man's abdomen.

- Go over the features described in Cases 44 and 45.
- Common to uncommon conditions:
  1. Hepatic cirrhosis with portal hypertension.
  2. Myeloproliferative conditions.
  3. Malignant lymphoma.
  4. Leukaemia.
  5. Right-sided heart failure.
  6. Constrictive pericarditis.
  7. Infiltrative conditions, e.g. sarcoidosis, amyloidosis.
  8. Infections (see Case 45).
  9. Budd–Chiari syndrome.
  10. Glycogen storage disorders.

Examiner

What causes of ascites do you know of?

Candidate

The causes are several and may be sub-divided according to the nature of the ascitic fluid, i.e. transudate, exudate, or chylous.

1. Causes of a transudate:
   a. Hepatic cirrhosis.
   b. Congestive cardiac failure.
   c. Nephrotic syndrome.
   d. Protein losing enteropathies.
2. Causes of an exudate:
   a. Malignancy.
      – Carcinoma (ovary, gut, secondaries, etc.)
   b. Infective.
      – Tuberculous.
      – Acute bacterial.

3. Causes of chylous fluid:
   a. Trauma.
   b. Malignancy.

CASE 47 RENAL ENLARGEMENT

General advice

When a mass in the left renal angle is felt, be sure that you go through the motions of distinguishing the kidney from the spleen (see Case 45 and Table below).

Do not forget that some patients with enlarged kidneys may have had a renal transplant. Look for a surgical scar and the presence of a mass in the pelvis (pelvic transplanted kidney).

Examiner

Examine this man's abdomen and tell me what the diagnosis is.

Locally

- Go on to examining the abdomen as described previously.
- Do not forget to palpate both kidneys.

Elsewhere

- Look for periorbital puffiness.
- Look for signs of uraemia.
- Examine for anaemia and pedal oedema.

Candidate

This undistressed young man has a soft non-distended, non-tender abdomen which on palpation revealed a mass in the left loin, which moved with respiration. I was able to palpate above and below this mass and it was ballotable. The mass, though smooth, was irregular in outline. No other organomegaly was found. There was no associated bruit.

Examiner

What are your differential diagnoses?

Candidate

1. Polycystic kidney disease.
2. Hydronephrosis.
3. Renal tumour.
4. Nephrotic syndrome.

The most likely diagnosis is that of polycystic disease of the kidneys. An alternative diagnosis might be that of renal cell carcinoma; however, the age of the patient makes this unlikely. Another potential cause is that of unilateral hydronephrosis; however, such kidneys tend to be smooth in contour.

Examiner

What investigations would you organize to confirm your clinical findings?

Candidate

Investigations that I would arrange for include:

1. A biochemical profile, FBC and ESR.
2. Examine the urine for blood and protein.
3. A renal ultrasound scan.
4. An intravenous pyelogram.
5. A renal angiogram.

Examiner

What can you tell me about polycystic kidney disease?

Candidate

Polycystic kidney disease has two forms, a so-called adult form that has an **autosomal dominant** pattern of inheritance and an infantile form that has an **autosomal recessive** pattern. The latter form is often fatal in childhood. The kidneys and also the liver are affected by multiple cysts that are responsible for the enlargement of one or both kidneys. Common manifestations in adults include haematuria (microscopic or macroscopic), hypertension, recurrent urinary tract infections and uraemia. Rarely, the condition may be so mild that the individual is asymptomatic, and the condition presents as an autopsy finding. There is an increased incidence of berry aneurysms and hence intra-cranial haemorrhages.

Differentiation of left kidney enlargement from splenomegaly

	Kidney	Spleen
Borders	Rounded	Sharp edge
Possible to pass palpating fingers between upper end of kidney and ribs	Yes	No
Bimanually palpable	Yes	No
Presence of colonic resonance on percussion anteriorly	Yes	No
Movement with respiration	Slightly	Freely

CASE 48 ASCITES

Examiner

Examine this patient's abdomen.

Locally

- Make sure the abdomen is fully exposed (above the groins and up to the nipples).
- Note the distended abdomen with distension in the flanks (remember to view the distension from the foot of the bed and go through the causes of abdominal swelling in your head (fat, fluid, flatus, fetus, faeces and organ enlargement).
- Inspect for any dilated veins over the abdominal wall and if present ascertain the direction of blood flow in them.
- Look for an everted umbilical hernia.
- Go over the abdominal examination routine.
- If liver or spleen enlargement is suspected, make sure that the examiner sees you going over the motions of demonstrating that you have carried out the tests to distinguish between spleen and kidney and have 'dipped' the liver in gross ascites and have percussed the upper border of the liver.
- Examine for a 'fluid thrill' and 'shifting dullness'.
- When the cause is not becoming obvious, think of causes other than liver, kidney, spleen enlargement for the clinical signs (ascites with or without an abdominal mass).

  - Intra-abdominal causes (nephrotic syndrome, abdominal TB, carcinomatosis, lymphomas).
  - Extra-abdominal causes (CCF, constrictive pericarditis).

Elsewhere

- Look for stigmata of liver cirrhosis (see Case 46)
- Look for signs of congestive cardiac failure or constrictive pericarditis (raised JVP and pedal and sacral oedema, etc.).
- Palpate the left supraclavicular gland.

Candidate

This patient has abdominal distension with fullness in the flanks and and everted umbilicus. (Go on to present all positive findings). These suggest the presence of ascites. (You can relate more information of possible aetiology if you have elicited the relevant signs.)

Examiner

What investigations would you like to perform?

Candidate

To confirm the diagnosis and then to ascertain the nature and aetiology of the ascites I would like to perform:

1. Abdominal ultrasound.
2. Ascitic fluid tap (protein, cytology, culture, and bacteriology including stain and culture for tubercle bacilli).

Note: Obviously you would list any relevant investigation if you had detected signs of liver cirrhosis; constrictive pericarditis; etc.

CASE 49 MASS IN THE EPIGASTRIUM

Examiner

Examine this patient's tummy.

Locally

On inspection from the foot of the bed the epigastric fullness will be detected.

- Look for visible peristalsis and movement with respiration.
- Go through the abdominal examination routine; make sure you define the consistency and size of the mass and try and differentiate this from an enlarged left lobe of the liver or an enlarged spleen.
- Points to go over when the epigastric mass is likely:

  – Check for gastric splash.
  – Check for expansibility or transmitted pulsations.
  – Look for fluid thrill which may be present in large pancreatic cysts.

- Listen to the bowel sounds.
- Listen for bruit over the mass.

Elsewhere

- Look for cachexia and jaundice (pancreatic tumour).
- Examine for left supraclavicular gland enlargement (carcinoma of the stomach).
- Anaemia?

Candidate

This patient has a mass in the epigastrium as evidenced by (give your signs and give negative or positive findings which may point towards aetiology).

What is the differential diagnosis of an epigastric mass?

Candidate

Five conditions have to be excluded:

1. Carcinoma of the stomach.
2. Carcinoma of the transverse colon.
3. Aneurysm of the abdominal aorta.
4. Pancreatic tumour or pseudocyst.
5. Retroperitoneal lymphadenopathy.

Examiner

What investigations would you request?

Candidate

1. Abdominal ultrasound.
2. Barium meal.
3. CT scan of the abdomen.
4. Endoscopy.

Examiner

How useful is the carcinoembryonic antigen in the diagnosis of carcinoma of the stomach?

Candidate

Elevation of the CEA levels is common in several tumours including GI tumours (stomach, colon, and pancreas), ovary, lung and breast. Rise in CEA levels can also occur when the tumour metastasizes and is not limited to GI tumours alone. Measuring CEA levels is probably more important for monitoring the progress of the tumours after treatment. Falling CEA levels are indicative of regression of tumour. Sometimes, pancreatitis, inflammatory bowel disease, cirrhosis and rectal polyps may cause mild elevations in CEA.

Discussion on mass in the epigastrium

Malignancies of the gastrointestinal tract (gastric, pancreatic and colonic cancers) are common conditions in the USA and Europe. An increased risk of GI malignancies occurs in patients with pernicious anaemia, ulcerative colitis and familial polyposis. Patients with gastric cancer usually present with anorexia, weight loss, upper abdominal discomfort and distension even after taking small meals. GI blood loss is common and sometimes the diagnosis of gastric cancer becomes apparent on barium meal/endoscopy while one is looking for the underlying cause for anaemia.

Histological confirmation of the diagnosis through endoscopic biopsy is essential. Although colonic cancer is most common in the rectosigmoid region, transverse colon may also be affected. Besides an epigastric mass, a patient with carcinoma of the transverse colon may present with anaemia and abdominal discomfort. A change in bowel habit is an early feature of the carcinoma if the descending colon is involved. Since the bowel contents remain liquid in patients with carcinoma of the ascending and transverse colon, features of obstruction and change of bowel habits are not common until the late stage.

Carcinoma of the head of the pancreas typically presents with nausea, anorexia, weight loss and progressive painless jaundice. With carcinoma of the body of the pancreas, the symptoms are often ill-defined and consist of vague upper abdominal pain that may be worse on lying down and may occasionally radiate to the back. The formation of a pseudocyst is a common complication of acute pancreatitis. The term pseudocyst is used since as compared to a true cyst a pseudocyst does not have an epithelial lining. The 'pseudo' cavity usually contains necrotic tissue, blood and pancreatic secretion and its walls are formed by surrounding structures.

CASE 50 MASS IN THE RIGHT ILIAC FOSSA

Examiner

Examine this patient's abdomen.

Locally

- Go through the inspection, palpation, percussion, auscultation routine.
- Look for any visible swelling.
- Look for any visible peristalsis.
- Check whether there are any skin sinuses.
- Palpate for masses apart from liver, spleen, kidney, and lymph nodes.
- Define the size, surface, consistency and tenderness of the mass.
- Auscultate for bowel sounds, bruits.

Elsewhere look for

- Anaemia.
- Lymphadenopathy.
- Clubbing (Crohn's disease).
- Pyoderma gangrenosum.

Candidate

This patient has an abdominal mass in the right iliac fossa as determined by (give your physical signs).

Examiner

What are the causes of a mass in the right iliac fossa?

Candidate

There are several differential diagnoses to keep in mind. These are:

1. Crohn's disease.
2. Appendicular mass.
3. Tubo-ovarian mass.
4. Carcinoid tumour.
5. Infectious causes: TB, amoeboma, schistosomiasis, actinomycosis.

Examiner

What five investigations would you ask for?

Candidate

1. Abdominal ultrasound.
2. Barium meal and follow through.
3. Colonoscopy and biopsy.
4. Stool examination for amoebic cysts/trophozoites.
5. Urinary 5-hydroxy-indole-acetic acid (5-HIAA) (carcinoid tumours).

Examiner

Name five foods that may cause an increase in 5-HIAA levels

Candidate

Some increase in 5-HIAA levels occur with ingestion of:

1. Chocolate.
2. Bananas.
3. Tomatoes.
4. Pineapples.
5. Walnuts.

Discussion on mass in the right iliac fossa

Crohn's disease is a chronic inflammatory bowel disorder of unknown aetiology that may involve any segment of the gastrointestinal tract from mouth to anus; the terminal ileum is most commonly affected. Symptoms include diarrhoea, nausea, weight loss, anaemia and low grade pyrexia. With chronic inflammation of the terminal ileum, thickened loops of bowel with mesenteric involvement may be felt as a mass in the right iliac fossa. In appendicitis, a right iliac fossa mass may be seen in up to 30% of cases. Bowel sounds are usually present unless there is perforation and diffuse peritonitis.

Tuberculosis of the alimentary tract is again emerging in the light of AIDS in the west and is quite common in the developing countries. The clinical features are indistinguishable from Crohn's. In the ileocaecal region, a mass may be palpable because of granulomatous infiltration and fibrosis. Patients respond well to anti-TB therapy.

Carcinoid syndrome is characterized by the presence of an enterochromaffin cell tumour most commonly affecting the ileum (sometimes other parts of the GI tract) and the bronchus or ovaries. The tumour secretes excessive amounts of vasoactive substances including serotonin, histamine, and bradykinin. Symptoms often result from distant metastases of the tumour. Abdominal mass and discomfort with diarrhoea are common. Asthma and wheezing and cutaneous flushing are not uncommon. Metastasis to the heart may cause right-sided valvular lesions (pulmonary stenosis and tricuspid regurgitation). Resection of tumour is the treatment of choice.

CASE 51 DILATED ABDOMINAL WALL VEINS

Examiner

Look at the abdomen and then carry out the relevant examination.

Locally

- The dilated and prominent veins around the umbilicus will be obvious.
- Go on to demonstrate the direction of flow of the blood in the veins (see discussion, below).
- Palpate for hepatosplenomegaly (see Case 46).
- Examine for ascites (see Case 48).

Elsewhere

- Look for signs of cirrhosis (see Case 46).

Candidate

This patient has dilated abdominal veins with signs of cirrhosis of the liver (go on to present all your positive findings).

Examiner

What are the dilated abdominal veins called?

Candidate

Caput medusae.

Examiner

What are the common causes of dilated abdominal veins?

1. Portal vein obstruction from any cause.
2. Inferior vena cava obstruction.

Examiner

Give three common causes of inferior vena cava obstruction.

Candidate

1. Trauma.
2. Tumour obstructing blood flow.
3. Thrombosis.

Examiner

What is the hepatorenal syndrome?

Candidate

Hepatorenal syndrome is said to exist when renal failure develops in a patient with cirrhosis and ascites. The decline in the kidney function is only secondary to liver failure; improvement in liver function is associated with improvement in renal function. The exact mechanism of this syndrome remains unclear. The onset of renal failure is accompanied by acute intrarenal vasoconstriction and reduction in the renal blood flow. Serum renin and aldosterone levels are typically high. The renal tubular functions remain normal; oliguria is common. Severe renal failure may develop over a period of days to weeks. In all cases, other underlying causes of renal failure must be excluded. There is no satisfactory treatment available. Plasma expansion with monitoring of renal output has been noted to be beneficial. Prognosis remains poor; over 90% of patients die, mostly because of progressive liver failure, hepatic encephalopathy or sepsis.

Discussion on dilated abdominal veins

Distended veins radiating from the umbilicus are called caput medusae. Portal obstruction resulting in the establishment of a connection between the portal and parietal veins by means of the round ligament is the explanation for these dilated veins. In a thin person with a significant degree of wasting, the veins may become unduly prominent over the abdominal wall. If the veins are significantly dilated, the findings assume greater clinical significance.

You must learn to practise demonstrating the direction of flow in these veins.

1. First express the blood from a dilated and prominent segment of the veins with two fingers by gentle pressure.
2. While maintaining the pressure, take off one of the fingers and notice how quickly the veins are filled with blood from the other end.
3. Now repeat the procedure (steps 1 and 2) but this time take off the pressure from the other end and compare whether the flow is greater upwards or downwards.

The direction in which the vein quickly refills is the direction of the blood flow.

In a normal healthy adult, the blood flow in the lower two-thirds of the abdominal wall is from above, downwards. Reversal of the blood flow commonly results from inferior vena caval obstruction. Because of the development of collateral circulation, the blood is carried to the superior vena cava via the collaterals seen in the form of the prominent veins on the abdomen.

PART 5

Central Nervous System

GENERAL ADVICE

Do not be put off by a case which requires examination of the CNS. These short cases will have obvious abnormalities which will be easily demonstrable. These cases are given to demonstrate your skills at examining the CNS competently and interpreting the signs reasonably.

Most CNS short cases centre around cranial nerve palsies, cerebellar lesions and spastic or flaccid lower limb paralysis.

Know the routes taken by the cranial nerves and the clinical conditions produced by lesions at various sites of the pathways.

For examination of ocular muscle movements remember that the lateral rectus is supplied by the 6th cranial nerve, the superior oblique by the 4th cranial nerve and the remaining ocular muscles by the 3rd cranial nerve (LR6, SO4 remainder 3).

Practice repeatedly examination of the cranial nerves (in healthy adults as well as in patients with pathology) up to a point that it becomes routine and will pose no problem in the exam.

Learn to recognize the facial appearance of common cranial nerve palsies.

CASE 52 PSEUDOBULBAR PALSY

Examiner

Examine this patient's cranial nerves.

Locally

- Go on to examine all cranial nerves in a systematic and methodical fashion.
- Note during the examination that the patient will have emotional lability (may have a peculiar facial expression or laugh and cry for no apparent reason).
- Do not forget to ask the patient to protrude the tongue (and say 'La, La, La'). Note that this can be performed by the patient only with difficulty because of spasticity and stiffness of the tongue.
- Test for movement of the soft palate (ask patient to say 'Kuh, Kuh, Kuh' with mouth open). The palate will be paralysed.
- Demonstrate the briskness of the jaw jerk.
- Test for dysarthria (ask patient for his address or ask him to repeat 'West Register Street').

Elsewhere

- Look for presence of fasciculations in the limb muscles (motor neurone disease).
- Look for upper motor neurone signs, usually more marked in the lower limbs with spasticity, brisk reflexes, and upgoing plantars.

Candidate

This patient has pseudobulbar palsy as evidenced by ... (go on to give your physical signs).

Examiner

Give me three causes of pseudobulbar palsy.

Candidate

1. Motor neurone disease.
2. Multiple sclerosis.
3. Bilateral cerebrovascular accidents.

Examiner

What is bulbar palsy?

Candidate

This condition is less common than pseudobulbar palsy. It is characterized by bilateral wasting of the tongue with fasciculation, paralysis of the palate, dysarthria, and, rarely, extraocular muscle palsy. The lesion is that of lower motor neurone type and may be caused by motor neurone disease or syringomyelia.

Examiner

What are the differences between bulbar and pseudobulbar palsy?

Candidate

Go through the table below.

	Bulbar palsy	*Pseudobulbar palsy*
Lesion site	Medulla oblongata	Cortical area
Lesion type	Lower motor neurone	Upper motor neurone
Paresis of the lip, tongue, pharynx, larynx	Yes	Yes
Swallowing difficulties with nasal regurgitation	Yes	Yes
Dysarthria	Yes	Yes
Tongue atrophy spasticity	Yes Flaccid	No Spastic

Discussion on pseudobulbar palsy

Pseudobulbar palsy is characterized by bilateral upper motor neurone (supranuclear) lesion of the 9th, 10th or 12th cranial nerves. The condition is not uncommon in elderly patients and is usually seen as a result of bilateral cortical involvement due to recurrent strokes. Spastic dysarthria occurs mainly because of the spasticity of the vocal cords; laryngeal nerve involvement may even lead to stridor. The tongue is spastic and can hardly be protruded. Both in bulbar as well as pseudobulbar palsy, nasal regurgitation of food and fluid may be troublesome and is seen because of paralysis of the soft palate and the pharyngeal muscles. Clonus of the lower jaw may be present because of the upper motor neurone lesion of the masseter muscles. A peculiar and rather fixed facial expression may be seen because of the spasticity of the facial muscles. The cause of emotional lability, a common feature of pseudobulbar palsy, remains unclear.

CASE 53 3RD CRANIAL NERVE PALSY

Examiner

Look at the patient's face and examine him/her appropriately.

Locally

- Note that the eyeball is rotated outwards (by the unopposed action of the lateral rectus) and downwards (by the unopposed action of the superior oblique). This will alert you to a cranial nerve palsy affecting the eye (3rd, 6th or 4th nerve palsy).
- Note the ptosis of the eyelid on the affected eye (due to drooping of the levator palpebrae superioris).
- Check the size of the pupils and test their reaction to light and accommodation (pupil is dilated because of 3rd nerve palsy leading to unopposed action of sympathetic impulses; and there is loss of light and accommodation reflexes).
- Demonstrate efficiently that the eyeball does not move in the direction controlled by the muscles supplied by the 3rd cranial nerve. The diplopia will increase in the direction of action of the paralysed muscle.

Candidate

This patient has a 3rd nerve palsy affecting the left eye as evidenced by ptosis, dilated pupil unresponsive to light and accommodation reflex, squint with the eyeball rotated downwards and outwards, and increasing diplopia and poor eyeball movements in the direction of action of eye muscles supplied by the 3rd cranial nerve.

Examiner

What is ptosis?

Candidate

Drooping of the eyelid is called ptosis. Normally only the upper one-sixth of the cornea is covered by the eyelid; anything more than that is called ptosis.

Examiner

Tell me something about the lesions affecting the 3rd cranial nerve during its course.

Candidate

Since the two nuclei lie close together, a nuclear lesion may affect both of the 3rd nerves and the ptosis is partial in these lesions. Multiple sclerosis, neoplasm or haemorrhage can affect the 3rd nerve at its origin. If the lesion is in the base of the midbrain it commonly causes 3rd nerve palsy with crossed hemiplegia due to involvement of the corticospinal tracts (Weber's syndrome). In the interpeduncular space, aneurysm at the junction of the posterior cerebral artery with the posterior communicating artery may compress the 3rd nerve. Further in its course, cavernous sinus lesions involve the 3rd nerve, the 4th nerve, and ophthalmic division of the 5th and 6th nerves. Fractures or retro-orbital swellings also involve the ophthalmic division of the 5th and 6th cranial nerves along with the 3rd nerve.

Discussion on 3rd cranial nerve palsy

The 3rd cranial nerve (oculomotor nerve) supplies the medial rectus, superior rectus and the inferior oblique muscles. In addition it supplies the pupilloconstrictor and levator palpebrae muscles. It is important to understand the exact role of the extraocular muscles in the movements of the eyeball. For example, if a patient with right-sided 3rd nerve palsy is asked to look straight, the right eye will turn laterally because of the unopposed action of the lateral rectus (supplied by the 6th nerve) and diplopia results. When the patient is asked to look to the far right, both eyes can move in the right direction. If the patient is asked to look to the far left, the right eye (with the 3rd nerve palsy) fails to cross the midline because of the failed action of the medial rectus and diplopia results.

Diplopia is an important clinical feature of 3rd nerve palsy. If the 3rd nerve lesion is due to an aneurysm, the pupillary dilatation is a prominent feature. In patients with diabetic neuropathy, the pupil is not dilated. In all patients with cranial nerve palsies, it is not only important to detect the cranial nerve lesion but also to find out through appropriate clinical examination and investigations (including CT and MRI) the underlying cause of the cranial neuropathy.

CASE 54 6TH NERVE (ABDUCENT) PALSY

Examiner

Look at the patient's face and examine him/her appropriately.

- A squint will be apparent.
- Notice the medial deviation of the affected eyeball (conferent squint: see Case 57). This is due to the unopposed action of the medial rectus muscle.
- Go on to quickly testing visual acuity (rule out blindness and the presence of a glass eye).
- Test the various movements of each eye methodically by testing eye movements in all directions.
- In cases of mild palsies, the patient will experience diplopia when moving the eye in the direction of the affected muscle, so, ask the patient whether he/she sees double with each movement!

Candidate

This patient has a right (or left) 6th nerve palsy as seen by medial deviation of the right eye and failure of the eyeball to move laterally with consequent diplopia.

Examiner

What is the lateral medullary syndrome?

Candidate

The lateral medullary syndrome (Wallenberg's syndrome) is characterized by the thrombosis of the vertebral or the posterior inferior cerebellar artery. The clinical features include:

1. Numbness and impaired sensation over the half of the face (ipsilateral 5th cranial nerve damage).
2. Loss of taste (nucleus and tractus solitarius).
3. Dysphasia, paralysis of vocal cords and hoarseness (9th and 10th nerves).

4. Ipsilateral cerebellar signs.
5. Ipsilateral Horner's syndrome (sympathetic fibres).
6. Vertigo, nystagmus, diplopia (vestibular nucleus).
7. Contralateral loss of pain and temperature over half of the body (spinothalamic tract).

Discussion on 6th nerve (abducent) palsy

The 6th cranial nerve (abducent nerve) originates in the pons. Since the nucleus of the 7th cranial nerve is also close by, a lesion of the pons may involve both the 6th and the 7th cranial nerves. The 6th cranial nerve has a long intracranial course and thus is commonly involved in pathology affecting the brain. It exits the brainstem and passes over the petrous bone before entering the cavernous sinus. The 3rd, 4th and 6th cranial nerves all pass through the cavernous sinus before entering the superior orbital fissure along with the sympathetic fibres serving the iris and eyelids. If the lesion is in the midbrain, the 3rd and 4th nerves are commonly affected with the 6th nerve.

Pontine lesions are most commonly associated with 6th cranial nerve palsy. Brainstem lesions that may affect the 6th cranial nerve include malignancy, vascular abnormalities and multiple sclerosis. All three cranial nerves mentioned (3rd, 4th and 6th) may also be affected by meningitis or carcinomatous infiltration of the meninges. During its course through the cavernous sinus and superior orbital fissure the nerves may be involved by: orbital tumour, cavernous sinus thrombosis, or aneurysm of the internal carotid artery. In most cases, an isolated 6th cranial nerve palsy results from microvascular ischaemia (especially in diabetic adults). In children a common cause is the post viral syndrome.

CASE 55 7TH CRANIAL NERVE (FACIAL) PALSY

Examiner

Look at the patient's face and then go on to examine her/him.

Locally

- The asymmetry of the face will be obvious.
- Note the loss of the nasolabial folds on one side.
- Go on to testing for all muscles supplied by the facial nerve using simple instructions such as (1) 'Show me your teeth', (2) 'Smile', (3) 'Blow out your cheeks', (4) 'Screw your eyes up tight and don't let me open them with my fingers', (5) 'Look up' or 'produce furrows on your forehead'.
- Distinguish between an upper motor neurone lesion and a lower motor neurone lesion (an upper motor neurone lesion will affect only the lower part of the affected side of the face; a lower motor neurone lesion affects a complete half of the face).
- Test for the corneal reflex (sensory supply by the 5th cranial nerve, but closing of eye by the 7th = orbicularis oculi).
- Ask for the presence of hyperacusis (stapedius muscle involvement).
- Ask for any change in taste or abnormal taste sensation (supplies anterior two-thirds of tongue).

Elsewhere

- If lesion is an upper motor type of facial palsy, look for the presence of associated hemiparesis since signs of stroke on the same side are often present, with or without speech difficulties.
- If lesion is of the lower motor neurone type look for:

  - Parotid swelling (tumour).
  - Scar of mastoid surgery (look behind ear).
  - Look at the nose for lupus pernio (sarcoid may cause bilateral facial palsy of lower motor neurone type).

Candidate

This patient has a 7th cranial nerve palsy of the lower motor neurone type (or upper motor neurone type as the case may be) as seen by the presence of . . . (go on to give your physical signs).

Examiner

What is the Ramsay Hunt syndrome?

Candidate

Ramsay Hunt syndrome is due to herpes zoster affecting the geniculate ganglion. It is a rare condition that is characterized by vertigo, hearing loss, pain in the ear and lower motor neurone facial palsy. Painful vesicles may also develop in the external auditory canal and the palate.

Examiner

What are the causes of a lower motor neurone 7th nerve palsy?

Candidate

Lesions can occur at several points of the pathway taken by the 7th cranial nerve. The causes at various points are:

1. In the pons at the origin of the nerve:

    – Vascular lesion.
    – Tumour.
    – Multiple sclerosis.

2. At the cerebellopontine angle:

    – Acoustic neuroma.

3. At the facial canal:

    – Middle ear infections.
    – Bell's palsy.

– Parotid gland tumour.
– Mastoid surgery.

Lower motor neurone lesions may also occur with any cause of peripheral neuropathy, e.g. sarcoidosis, leprosy.

Discussion on 7th cranial nerve (facial) palsy

The facial nerve (7th cranial nerve) supplies the muscles of facial expression, the stapedius muscle, and is responsible for the taste sensation from the anterior two-thirds of the tongue. Parasympathetic motor fibres to the salivary glands and chorda tympani are also carried with the facial nerve. Since a minor degree of facial asymmetry is not uncommon, one should not jump into making a diagnosis of facial nerve palsy without a thorough examination revealing the presence of definitive physical signs. The most common cause for an upper motor neurone lesion is a stroke that is characterized by weakness of the lower face contralateral to the lesion. The upper face is spared because of the bilateral innervation.

If the lesion is of the lower motor neurone type, there is total involvement of the ipsilateral facial muscles. A lower motor neurone lesion may result from lesions at any point between the origin of the nerve from the nucleus right through to the site of supply, i.e. facial muscles (see above). Bilateral symmetrical weakness of the facial muscles is produced by muscle dystrophies such as myasthaenia gravis and myotonic dystrophy.

Bell's palsy is characterized by a sudden and unilateral weakness of the facial muscles of the lower motor neurone type. The precise cause of this condition is unknown but it is thought to result because of the swelling of the nerve in the narrow part of the petrous bone during its course through the facial canal. Post-auricular pain may precede the actual weakness of the facial muscles. Decreased lacrimation, abnormal taste sensation and hyperacusis may also be present. Almost all patients with partial facial nerve palsy have a complete recovery within 3–6 months. With complete paralysis, 10–20% of patients may be left with residual weakness. Some patients develop synkinetic movements characterized by winking of the eyes upon chewing. Excessive lacrimation is also a recognized complication.

Steroid therapy (prednisolone 60–80 mg/day for 5–7 days followed by a reduction of dose to 10–20 mg per day with weaning off within two weeks) may be beneficial. Early steroid therapy (within 24 hours of onset) is thought to reduce the oedema and may result in early recovery and a lower incidence of complications. Some physicians advocate acyclovir in addition to steroids (Bell's was thought to be due to herpes). Persistent facial muscle weakness may require hypoglossal–facial nerve anastomosis.

CASE 56 EXOPHTHALMOS (PROPTOSIS)

Examiner

Look at the patient and then examine him appropriately.

Locally

- Note the undue prominence of the eyeball ('stare').
- Observe the patient in profile from above the head.
- Look for lid retraction and wide palpebral fissures.
- Test for presence of lid lag (with your finger two feet away from the eyes ask the patient to follow your finger as you slowly move the finger up and then down. The eyelids lag behind the movement of the rest of the eye showing quite a bit of the sclera).
- Look for corneal oedema.
- Check for eyeball movements to rule out exophthalmic ophthalmoplegia.
- Listen with your stethoscope over the eyeballs for bruit.

Elsewhere

- Examine for thyroid enlargement in the neck.
- Check for presence of fine tremors of the fingers (ask the patient to outstretch hands with fingers wide apart and place a piece of A4-sized paper on them if the tremor is not obvious).
- Examine for sweaty palms and thyroid acropachy (clubbing-like changes in nails).
- Feel pulse for atrial fibrillation.
- Look at the legs and feel for pretibial myxoedema.
- Ask examiner for permission to examine the cardiovascular system.

Candidate

This patient has exophthalmos (say whether it is unilateral or bilateral) which is most likely due to (give your most likely diagnosis. The physical signs present are ... (go on to give your findings, positive and negative).

Examiner

What are the causes of unilateral exophthalmos?

Candidate

There are several causes:

1. Thyrotoxicosis (early stage).
2. Retro-orbital cellulitis.
3. Cavernous sinus thrombosis (usually seen with chemosis and ophthalmoplegia).
4. Arterio-venous aneurysm.
5. Leukaemic infiltration or granuloma.
6. Retro-orbital tumours (Burkitt's lymphoma or retino-blastoma).

Examiner

What is Graves' disease?

Candidate

Grave's disease is a term given to a clinical triad which comprises clinical features of:

1. Thyrotoxicosis.
2. Goitre.
3. Pretibial myxoedema.

Examiner

How is progressive exophthalmos treated?

Candidate

Medical and surgical measures are available:

1. Medical measures include:
   a. Sunglasses to protect eyes from dust and foreign bodies.
   b. Methyl cellulose eye drops to prevent corneal dryness.
   c. Diuretics to reduce orbital oedema.
   d. Steroids in high doses.
2. Surgical measures:
   a. Tarsorrhaphy.
   b. Orbital decompression.

Discussion on exophthalmos

Exophthalmos or proptosis is characterized by a staring expression with prominence of the eyeballs and retraction of the upper eyelids. Hyperthyroidism is a common cause of exophthalmos. Although in most patients with hyperthyroidism the condition is bilateral, in the early stages, exophthalmos may be more marked in one eye. Exophthalmos may also develop in an eye of a patient previously treated for hyperthyroidism. Beside lid retraction, lid lag and wide palpebral fissures are important physical signs that usually result because of excessive sympathetic stimulation. Infiltrative ophthalmopathy occurs due to what is thought to be auto-immune disease. Retro-orbital fat, connective tissue, and the muscles are all involved.

With progressive protrusion, the patient may have difficulty in closing the eyelids. Exposure of the cornea may lead to corneal ulceration. Besides the clinical impression, exophthalmos and its progression must be measured by use of an exophthalmoscope. CT scan can also demonstrate the ocular muscle involvement and retro-orbital masses. Increasing intraorbital pressure requires urgent surgical attention.

CASE 57 SQUINT

Examiner

Examine this patient's eyes.

- The squint will be obvious and thus examination of the eye must quickly focus on distinguishing a paralytic from a non-paralytic squint.
- Full examination of the ocular movements of each eye separately is mandatory.
- Do not forget to ask the patient whether he/she sees double with every movement of the eye in the direction of action of the ocular muscles being tested.
- Once examination is complete, the answer should be precise.
- To identify the presence of a squinting eye use the cover test (the patient is asked to fix the eyes on an object. One eye is then covered and the movement of the other eye is observed. If the uncovered eye makes a movement to take up a fixation point then a squint is present). The test is repeated with the opposite eye. The fixing eye will not move when the squinting eye is covered.

Candidate

This patient has a non-paralytic squint affecting the right (or left) eye.

Examiner

What are the various muscle actions on the eyeball?

Candidate

The external rectus muscle which is supplied by the 6th cranial nerve abducts the eye. (Go through the list given in the Table below).

Examiner

What is the most common cause of a concomitant squint?

Candidate

An uncorrected error of refraction in early childhood is usually the cause. In concomitant squint the image from the defective eye is suppressed by the brain. In most cases, despite the use of suitable glasses, patients are left with a latent squint that becomes manifest during periods of fatigue and high fever often associated with systemic illnesses.

Discussion on squint

Squint or strabismus is a deviation of the eye from the normal optical axis.

Convergent squint is when the eye is deviated towards the nasal side while **divergent** squint is when the eye is deviated towards the temporal side.

When you are dealing with a case of squint you will have to decide whether you are dealing with an **incomitant/non-concomitant (paralytic)** or **concomitant (non-paralytic)** squint.

Paralytic (incomitant/non-concomitant) squint results from paralysis of one or more ocular muscles which is a consequence of lesions of the 3rd, 4th or 6th cranial nerves. Squints due to these nerve palsies are characterized by limitation of the eye movement in the direction of action of the respective eye muscle and by increasing diplopia in the direction of action of the muscle.

With **concomitant (non-paralytic)** squint there is muscle imbalance, but the ocular movements are full and the squint may be convergent or divergent.

Ocular axes: In concomitant (non-paralytic) squints the relationship between the two ocular axes remains constant in all directions while in incomitant (paralytic) squints the axes vary.

Image separation: In a patient with incomitant (paralytic) squint the separation of the images is maximum when the patient attempts to use the paralysed muscle by moving the eyeball in the direction controlled by the affected muscles.

An eye affected by concomitant (non-paralytic) squint is called 'lazy eye'.

Actions and nerve supply of the eyeball muscles

Muscle	Nerve supply	Action
External rectus	6th cranial nerve	Abduction
Internal rectus	3rd cranial nerve	Adduction
Superior oblique	4th cranial nerve	Depression when eye turned inwards
Inferior oblique	3rd cranial nerve	Elevation when eye turned inwards
Superior rectus	3rd cranial nerve	Elevation when eye turned outwards
Inferior rectus	3rd cranial nerve	Depression when eye turned outwards

CASE 58 NYSTAGMUS

Examiner

Examine this patient's eyes.

- Remember to hold your examining finger at least two feet away from the patient and not to go to the extreme left or right, i.e. beyond the range of binocular vision. If the testing finger is held close to the patient's eye a slight transient nystagmus is often seen and is not pathological.
- Determine whether the nystagmus is **pendular** (oscillations are equal in speed and amplitude in both directions) or **jerky** (quick and slow phases of the unequal direction).
- The quicker phase of the nystagmus is arbitrarily used to define the direction of nystagmus.
- If the nystagmus is pendular, check the visual acuity and look for features of conditions commonly responsible for this type of nystagmus, e.g. albinism; diseases of the retina causing poor vision (examine the fundus).
- If the nystagmus is jerky (more common type), determine whether the nystagmus is horizontal or vertical. Vertical nystagmus is usually a sign of brainstem disease.
- The slow phase of the nystagmus is on the diseased side in vestibular lesions (check for deafness with permission from examiner).
- Acoustic neuroma causes a horizontal nystagmus.
- Phasic nystagmus is seen in alcoholism and barbiturate poisoning.
- **Down beat** nystagmus is a rarity caused by lesions around the foramen magnum.
- When a cerebellar lesion is suspected, look for other cerebellar signs (intention tremor; scanning speech, disdiadokokinesis and hypotonia of the limbs).

Candidate

This patient has nystagmus (please state jerky or pendular) as evidenced by involuntary rhythmic oscillation of the eyes.

Examiner

What is dissociated or ataxic nystagmus?

Candidate

Ataxic nystagmus exists when the nystagmus is seen in the abducted eye only. If bilaterally present it is considered to be pathognomonic of multiple sclerosis.

Examiner

What are the causes of nystagmus?

Candidate

Nystagmus can occur due to several conditions:

1. Congenital.
2. Cerebellar disease.
3. Brainstem lesions.
4. 3rd, 4th or 6th cranial nerve lesions.
5. Vestibular disease.
6. Due to drugs, e.g., alcohol, phenytoin, phenobarbital, diazepam.

CASE 59 HORNER'S SYNDROME

Examiner

Look at this patient's face and carry out the appropriate examination (or)
Examine this patient's eyes.

Locally, note the following features

- The partial ptosis on either side.
- The small size of the pupil non-responsive to light on the same side as the ptosis.
- Enophthalmos.
- Anhydrosis (lack of sweating on the same side of the face; difficult to demonstrate but could come up in the discussion).

Elsewhere look for

- Eyes: look for nystagmus (brainstem lesion).
- Signs of apical lung lesion (clubbing; crackles; wasting of the first dorsal interosseus muscle of the hand on the side of the Horner's lesion. The muscle is supplied by T_1 which is commonly involved in apical lung lesions).
- Neck: cervical ribs; lymphadenopathy or scar of injury or operation.
- Upper limbs: check for evidence of patchy loss of sensation which occurs in syringomyelia.

Examiner

What are the causes of Horner's syndrome?

Candidate

Any lesion affecting the sympathetic supply results in Horner's syndrome. There are several causes, both congenital and acquired:

1. Lesions of the brainstem or cerebral hemisphere paralysing the autonomic pathways (infarction; pontine glioma; lateral medullary syndrome; coning of the temporal lobe).

2. Cervical cord lesions (C_8–T_1 lesions), e.g. syringomyelia, cord tumour.
3. Lesions in the superior mediastinum (T_1 lesion), e.g. aneurysm; glandular enlargement; bronchial carcinoma; apical TB; trauma to brachial plexus.
4. Neck lesions (sympathetic chain lesions), e.g. trauma; lymphadenopathy; neoplastic infiltration; cervical sympathectomy; post-neck surgery.

Examiner

What are the causes of a dilated pupil?

Candidate

Common causes of a dilated pupil include:

1. Mydriatic eye drops (atropine/homatropine).
2. 3rd cranial nerve lesion (absent or sluggish light and accommodation responses).
3. Sympathetic overactivity.
4. 2nd cranial nerve lesion, e.g. optic atrophy (direct light and accommodation reflex absent but consensual reflexes are intact).
5. Myotonic pupil (Holmes Adie pupil) seen commonly in young women; is usually unilateral; slow reaction to bright light; incomplete constriction to convergence; often associated with decreased or absent tendon reflexes.

CASE 60 PTOSIS

Examiner

Examine this patient's eyes (or)
Look at the patient's face and examine appropriately.

- Note the drooping of the upper eyelid(s).
- Determine whether the ptosis is:
  1. Unilateral or bilateral.
  2. Partial or complete.
  3. With or without overaction of the frontalis muscle.
- Look for presence of squint 3rd nerve palsy (or Horner's syndrome).
- Examine size of pupil (Horner's syndrome = small/miosis; while 3rd nerve palsy = dilated/mydriasis).
- Test light and accommodation reflexes.
- Look for evidence of myopathy and other features of dystrophia myotonica (cataract; frontal baldness; talk about excluding gonadal atrophy if this diagnosis is likely).

Examiner

What are the causes of ptosis?

Candidate

There are several causes of ptosis:

A. Congenital.

   This is a common cause of bilateral or unilateral ptosis with overaction of frontalis.

B. Acquired.

   1. 3rd nerve palsy (ptosis is usually unilateral with overaction of the frontalis; ptosis is complete or partial depending on the severity of involvement; pupil is dilated and a paralytic squint is present).
   2. Sympathetic paralysis (Horner's syndrome – see case 59). Ptosis is partial.

3. Tabes dorsalis (ptosis is usually bilateral with over-action of the frontalis).
4. Myopathies (e.g. fascioscapulohumeral myopathy; myotonic dystrophy; myasthaenia gravis).
5. Local lesions on the eyelid (e.g. hordeolum/stye/sebaceous cyst). Ptosis is unilateral and partial.
6. Hysterical ptosis is very rare and is unilateral.

CASE 60 ARGYLL ROBERTSON PUPILS (AR PUPILS)

Examiner

Examine this patient's eyes.

Locally

- Go through the routine of eye examination.
- Note carefully the size and regularity of the pupils (small, irregular and unequal).
- Do not forget to elicit the light and accommodation reflexes (the pupils are unresponsive to light: both direct and consensual light reflexes absent, but they respond to accommodation = convergence).
- Ptosis may accompany AR pupils.

Request examiner's permission to look for physical signs.

Elsewhere:

- Look for signs of aortic regurgitation.
- Examine for loss of proprioception with positive Romberg's sign.

Candidate

This patient has an incomplete ptosis, small irregular unequal pupils which do not react to light but do so to convergence. These signs are consistent with the Argyll Robertson pupils. In addition there are signs of aortic regurgitation and loss of proprioception with a positive Romberg's sign.

Examiner

What is a Holmes Adie pupil?

Candidate

This is a condition confined to women, always unilateral, where the pupil is larger than normal with an absent light reflex and very slow accommodation reflex. It is often associated with diminished or absent tendon reflexes.

Examiner

Name five conditions which may result in the AR type of pupils.

Candidate

The features of AR pupils may be seen in the following conditions:

1. Tertiary syphilis.
2. Diabetes mellitus.
3. Orbital injury.
4. Hereditary neuropathies.
5. Sarcoidosis.

Discussion on Argyll Robertson pupils

Although in your practice of clinical medicine you may have seen only a few patients with AR pupils, it is not uncommon to see such patients as short cases in the MRCP examination. The exact site of lesion in these patients is not known but it is thought to be the ciliary ganglion. The four important characteristics of AR pupils are:

1. Bilateral, small, irregular and unequal pupils.
2. There may be associated atrophy and depigmentation of the iris.
3. Pupils fail to react to light but accommodation reflex is retained.
4. Pupils fail to dilate properly in response to mydriatic drugs.

The above four features are almost diagnostic of neurosyphilis although many of the features may occur in diabetes mellitus, orbital injury, hereditary neuropathies and in sarcoidosis.

CASE 62 HOMONYMOUS HEMIANOPIA

Examiner

Examine this patient's visual fields.

- Sit about a half-metre distant, opposite the patient who is seated upright.
- Keep your eyes at about the same level as those of the patient.
- Ask whether the patient can see your finger ('how many fingers can you see') to quickly find out whether the patient is blind or not in that eye.
- Go on to test the field of vision in each eye separately and in every direction of the visual field.

    1. For testing the right eye ask the patient to cover his left eye with his left hand; you should cover/close your right eye to compare your visual field with that of the patient; thus you should be looking steadily in the patient's right eye with your left eye.
    2. Use a pin with a large head (e.g. hat pin). Check the extent of the peripheral visual fields by bringing the pin held in your left hand into the field of vision from the periphery at several points on the circumference. Examine from all quadrants so as to be sure about the complete field of vision on that side. Do not forget to examine for loss of visual field in the centre as well (scotoma).
    3. Now similarly examine the field of vision of the other eye. Ask the patient to cover his right eye with his right hand and you should now make sure that you transfer the pin to your right hand and you use your left hand to cover your left eye.

- Once you have diagnosed homonymous hemianopia you should go on to localize the lesion. Proceed to check the light reflex as well (if absent the lesion is between the optic chiasma and the midbrain but if the light reflex is present the lesion is placed between the midbrain and the occipital lobe).

Candidate

This patient has homonymous hemianopia.

Examiner

Where is the lesion?

Candidate

Since the light reflex is preserved the lesion lies between the midbrain and the occipital lobe.

Examiner

What is tunnel vision?

Candidate

Visual field defects are common in patients with optic atrophy irrespective of the underlying cause. Following papilloedema, for example, it is common to find that the blind spot is enlarged and the peripheral field of vision has constricted; a condition like retinitis pigmentosa may also be associated with marked constriction of visual field. In organic diseases, constricted visual field enlarges as the distance between the test object and the patient increases. If the constriction of visual field does not change with the distance of the visual test stimulus from the eye, it is often referred to as 'tunnel vision'. Tunnel vision may be seen in conditions like hysteria where there are no abnormal findings on fundoscopy.

Discussion on homonymous hemianopia

The optic nerve contains both the visual and pupillary fibres. The left and right optic nerves join at the optic chiasma and then where the visual fibres cross to join the uncrossed fibres to form the optic tract which travels to the geniculate body.

The optic radiation arising from the geniculate body travels to the visual cortex of the occipital lobe.

Testing of the visual fields is done to assess the type of lesion in the visual pathways. Clinical testing is very crude and usually finer assessment is done by perimetry.

Complete loss of vision (total blindness) in one eye may result from disease of the eye or a lesion of the optic nerve.

Hemianopia simply means an absence of one half of the visual field. Lateral hemianopia is more common than superior or inferior hemianopia.

Homonymous hemianopia indicates that the half loss of visual fields has affected similar fields in both eyes. For example, if the patient has right homonymous hemianopia, it means that he cannot see objects in the right half of the fields of both eyes.

Heteronymous hemianopia is rare but if present it would mean that the loss of field of vision is of the dissimilar halves on the two sides.

Quadrantic hemianopia is the loss of visual field in one quadrant of the field of vision.

The most common type of patient seen in the MRCP examination is one with stroke and homonymous hemianopia. It is important to be familiar with the three different sites of lesion in the visual pathways as listed below:

1. Optic nerve lesion resulting in blindness of the affected eye.
2. A lesion at the optic chiasma resulting in bitemporal hemianopia (pituitary and suprasellar tumours). Binasal hemianopia is extremely rare because it can result only if the uncrossed optic fibres on each side are affected by two separate lesions.
3. A lesion of the optic tract typically produces homonymous hemianopia (nasal field of one eye and the temporal field of the other eye).

CASE 63 CENTRAL SCOTOMA

Examiner

Examine this patient's visual fields.

- Thoroughly examine the field of vision (see Case 62).
- Once you have decided about the presence of a central scotoma, look into the fundus with your ophthalmoscope for any temporal pallor of the disc and other evidence of optic atrophy.

Candidate

This patient has a central scotoma (plus give any fundal findings you may see).

Examiner

What are the common causes of a central scotoma?

Candidate

The common causes of a central scotoma are:

1. Retrobulbar neuritis, most commonly in cases of multiple sclerosis.
2. Choroidoretinitis.
3. Pressure on the optic nerve by a tumour.
4. Optic atrophy due to toxins or vitamin B12 deficiency.

Examiner

What are the causes of sudden monocular blindness?

Candidate

Sudden loss of vision in one eye may result from:

1. Trauma to the eye.

2. Acute glaucoma.
3. Migraine.
4. Vascular causes (central retinal artery or central retinal vein occlusion; temporal arteritis).
5. Vitreous haemorrhage.
6. Retinal detachment.

Discussion on central scotoma

Scotomas are isolated small areas of loss of visual field.

Central scotomas result from the lesions in the macular areas.

Paracentral scotomas are seen as a result of lesions of the areas in close proximity to the macula and are commonly seen in early chronic simple glaucoma.

Peripheral scotomas are said to exist when isolated loss of vision is in the peripheral field.

In most cases the patient may not be aware of the isolated loss of vision and the defect may be noted only when the field of vision is tested by a physician. In contrast with peripheral scotomas, central scotomas are readily noticed because they affect the vision and result in the loss of visual acuity. Sometimes the terms negative and positive scotomas are used.

Negative scotomas are simply blind spots in the field of vision.

Positive scotomas are black or coloured light spots in some areas of the field of vision seen as scintillating flashes by the patient (commonly seen in migraine).

PART 6

Looking at the Fundi

GENERAL ADVICE

You may be asked to look at the fundus and in a short case you should be able to recognize the presence of papilloedema and in this case to look for the various stages as outlined below. You may also be asked to look at the fundus of a diabetic or hypertensive patient and to describe background retinopathy in diabetes and the various grades of retinal changes that occur in hypertension.

CASE 64 PAPILLOEDEMA

Examiner

Examine the patient's fundi (or)
Look at the fundi.

- It may suffice if you can recognize papilloedema.
- Do not forget to look at both fundi unless you are told specifically to look at the right or left fundus.
- Look for other fundal pathology (exudates, haemorrhages, choroidoretinitis).
- Try and identify the different stages of papilloedema:

    - Engorgement of the retinal veins.
    - Blurring of the disc margins.
    - A redder disc with loss of physiological cupping.

Candidate

This patient has papilloedema (in the right, left or both fundi) as evidenced by . . . (give your findings).

Examiner

What are the causes of papilloedema?

Candidate

There are several causes:

1. Raised intracranial pressure due to:

    - Intracranial mass lesions.
    - Encephalitis.
    - Trauma.
    - Subarachnoid haemorrhage.

2. Malignant hypertension.
3. Central retinal vein thrombosis.
4. Optic neuritis/papillitis.
5. Metabolic causes.
    - Hypercapnia.

– Hypoparathyroidism/hypocalcaemia.
– Chronic hypoxia.

6. Benign intracranial hypertension.

Examiner

What is pseudopapilloedema?

Candidate

In true papilloedema the physiological cup is well preserved until a late stage. Occasionally in certain conditions such as hypermetropia, there may be loss of physiological cupping and blurring of disc margins; these changes may mimic papilloedema and hence the term pseudopapilloedema.

Examiner

How is papillitis different from papilloedema?

Candidate

Papillitis is usually unilateral with loss of visual acuity whereas in papilloedema the condition is usually bilateral and the visual acuity remains normal although an enlargement of the blind spot occurs.

Examiner

What is the Foster Kennedy syndrome?

Candidate

This syndrome is characterized by papilloedema in one eye and optic atrophy in the other. This may be caused by a tumour of the frontal lobe which may cause optic atrophy because of the pressure on the optic nerve. With increase in the size of the tumour, there is a rise in the intracranial pressure and this causes papilloedema on the other side.

Discussion on papilloedema

Papilloedema means swelling of the optic disc (papilla). The earliest fundoscopic findings include engorgement of the retinal veins with loss of spontaneous pulsation. Redness of the disc with blurring and heaping up of its margins with eventual loss of the physiological cupping follows. This is a result of raised intracranial pressure resulting in pressure in the subarachnoid space around the optic nerves.

Malignant hypertension: the presence of papilloedema is essential for the diagnosis of malignant hypertension (in most cases retinal haemorrhages and exudates are also present). Papilloedema is also common in patients with hypertensive encephalopathy.

Brain tumours, abscesses, cysts: raised intracranial pressure with impaired venous return results in papilloedema.

The presence of papilloedema is considered to be a contra-indication for lumbar puncture since sudden release of CSF due to raised intracranial pressure may cause acute herniation of the cervical cord through the foramen magnum (pressure cone).

CASE 65 OPTIC ATROPHY

Examiner

Examine this patient's fundi.

- Note the pallor of the optic disc. A pale disc signifies optic atrophy.
- Look for evidence of papilloedema (disc contour, cup and cribrosa).
- Look for attenuation of veins and arterioles.

Candidate

This patient has optic atrophy in the left eye.

Examiner

What is consecutive optic atrophy?

Candidate

Optic atrophy resulting as a consequence of disease within the eye causing optic nerve damage is termed 'consecutive optic atrophy'. Some classifications include consecutive optic atrophy as part of secondary optic atrophy.

Examiner

What is Leber's optic atrophy?

Candidate

Leber's optic atrophy is a familial condition that primarily affects males. Clinical features include progressive visual loss, usually appearing in the second or third decades of life. On fundoscopic examination, at least in the early stages, there is evidence of oedema of the disc. After the acute stage is over the disc atrophy becomes well established. There is no satisfactory treatment available.

How do you distinguish primary from secondary optic atrophy?

There are several differing features of each type of atrophy (go through the list below).

Differences between primary and secondary optic atrophy

	Primary	*Secondary*
Preceding papilloedema	No	Yes
Disc contour, cup and cribrosa	Well circumscribed	Ill defined
Veins and arterioles	Attenuated	Arteries attenuated but veins congested
Causes	Multiple sclerosis Vitamin B12 deficiency Diabetes mellitus Toxic–tobacco, methyl alcohol, quinine Familial cerebellar ataxia	Brain tumour Temporal arteritis Thrombosis of central retinal artery

CASE 66 DIABETIC FUNDUS

Examiner

Examine the left fundus (or)
Examine the left eye.

- Look for changes of diabetic eye disease:

  - Rubeosis iridis (new vessel formation on iris).
  - Signs of 6th nerve palsy.
  - Cataracts.

- Background retinopathy changes:

  - Microaneurysms.
  - Tortuous and congested veins.
  - Dot and blot haemorrhages.
  - Exudates (usually 'hard' and 'waxy' with well defined edges).

- Proliferative retinopathy changes:

  - Neovascularization, i.e. new vessel formation over the disc and the nerves. Macular oedema may also accompany:
  - Pre-retinal haemorrhages.
  - Subhyaloid haemorrhages (boat-shaped vitreous haemorrhages).
  - Retinal detachment.

Candidate

This patient has diabetic retinopathy as evidenced by the following changes ... (list them).

Examiner

Are microaneurysms pathognomonic of diabetic retinopathy?

Candidate

No, besides diabetes mellitus, microaneurysms may also be seen in:

- Hypertension.
- Severe anaemia.
- Collagen vascular disease.
- Dysproteinaemia.

Examiner

What treatment is available for proliferative retinopathy?

Candidate

Photocoagulation or pituitary ablation.

Examiner

What diabetic changes can occur in the eye lens?

Candidate

Reversible osmotic changes (cause blurring of vision) and eventually cataract formation.

Discussion on diabetic fundus

Diabetic retinopathy remains a leading cause of blindness in adults. Most patients are over the age of 55 years and have had diabetes for over 10 to 15 years. Although there is a preponderance of retinopathy in those with poor blood glucose control there is no direct correlation of diabetic control with the incidence or severity of retinopathy. The two main types of diabetic retinopathy are:

1. Background or non-proliferative retinopathy.
2. Proliferative retinopathy.

Background retinopathy has also been called 'benign retinopathy' because many patients continue to have a fair degree of visual acuity despite the presence of background retinopathy.

Proliferative retinopathy is almost always associated with serious consequences including sudden blindness, thus proliferative retinopathy is referred to as 'malignant retinopathy'.

Pre-proliferative retinopathy is a term limited to those patients who have poor blood sugar control and have a rapid course of deterioration and blindness due to multiple areas of haemorrhage and exudate. In most cases diabetic patients with retinopathy also have co-existing neuropathy and nephropathy.

Microaneurysms are the earliest findings of background retinopathy and these are seen as well-defined areas of dilatation of the small retinal capillaries. Dot haemorrhages may be difficult to distinguish from microaneurysms. Tell the examiner that haemorrhages are usually irregular and disappear within a few days whereas microaneurysms are well-defined and last for months to years.

Exudates

1. Soft 'cotton wool' exudates are discreet areas of yellowish white patches that result from infarction of the inner layers of the retina.
2. Hard 'waxy' exudates are well-defined areas and are thought to be lipid deposits (see also Case 67).

Neovascularization is the presence of new blood vessel formation and results as a consequence of local ischaemia around the optic nerve.

Proliferative retinopathy is usually far worse in diabetic patients who continue to smoke and have co-existing hypertension.

CASE 67 HYPERTENSIVE FUNDUS

Examiner

Examine the fundus of the right eye.

Look for the various grades of retinopathy commonly known as the Keith Wagener changes.

- Grade I   Irregularity of the lumen of arteriole with increased tortuosity and increased light reflex (silver wiring).
- Grade II   Grade I changes above plus arteriovenous nipping.
- Grade III   Grade II changes above plus haemorrhages (most commonly flame-shaped) and exudates (hard and soft).
- Grade IV   Grade III changes above plus papilloedema.

Candidate

This patient has the following abnormalities in the fundus (list them). They suggest hypertensive retinopathy (state what grade if you are confident).

Examiner

Tell me something about retinal exudates.

Candidate

The 'soft' cotton wool exudates are due to poorly demarcated superficial ischaemic areas of necrosis of the retina or localized collections of oedema fluid in the nerve fibre layers. The presence of exudates may indicate the onset of an accelerated or malignant phase of hypertension. The exudates may disappear within a few weeks with good control of hypertension. 'Hard' exudates are small, deep and dense deposits of lipids and have well defined borders. They persist much longer than soft exudates.

Examiner

What are the important causes of retinal exudates?

Candidate

The important causes of exudates are:

1. Hypertension.
2. Diabetes mellitus.
3. Systemic lupus erythematosus.
4. Severe anaemia.
5. Leukaemia.

Discussion on hypertensive fundus

The retinal changes of hypertension reveal the severity of vascular damage that results from high pressure. The early changes of grade I, listed above, may also occur in atherosclerosis, even without hypertension. Grade III and grade IV changes are, of course, quite significant. Haemorrhagic areas are typically flame-shaped and may sometimes form a star around the macula (macular star).

Both soft and hard exudates may be seen in hypertension. The presence of papilloedema with raised blood pressure indicates malignant hypertension that requires urgent treatment. It is important to note that haemorrhage and exudates may be seen in hypertension as well as in diabetes mellitus. In many cases the same patient has hypertension as well as diabetes mellitus.

CASE 68 CHOROIDORETINITIS

Examiner

Look at this patient's left/right fundus.

- Go through the routine of fundal examination (optic disc, vessels, exudates, choroid and retina).
- Note the exudates appearing as white opaque areas of varying sizes surrounded by a black pigmented margin. The retinal vessels are always superficial to the exudates.
- Make a mental note of the size and number of these lesions and their location according to quadrants.
- Photocoagulation scars appear as choroidoretinitis and the changes of diabetic retinopathy will help distinguish them.

Candidate

This patient has several areas of choroidoretinitis dispersed in all quadrants of the retina (or has one localized area of choroidoretinitis in the upper nasal half of the retina).

Examiner

What are the causes of choroidoretinitis?

Candidate

There are several causes of choroidoretinitis:

1. Infective causes:

    TB, leprosy, toxoplasmosis, toxocariasis, syphilis, brucellosis, onchocerciasis.
2. Non-infective causes:

    Sarcoidosis, trauma, photocoagulation, retinitis pigmentosa.

Examiner

List four investigations which may help make a diagnosis.

Candidate

1. Chest X-ray.
2. Sabin and Feldman toxoplasma dye test.
3. Syphilis serology.
4. Serum angiotensin converting enzyme (SACE) levels or gallium lung scan.
5. Toxocara serology.
6. Eosinophilia.
7. Skin biopsy (leprosy and onchocerciasis).

Discussion on choroidoretinitis

The choroid is the vascular layer of the eye extending from the optic nerve posteriorly to the ciliary body anteriorly. Together with the iris and ciliary body the choroid constitutes the middle layer of the eye. The retina overlies the choroid. Inflammation of the choroid inevitably affects the retina and thus the term choroidoretinitis.

Acute suppurative choroidoretinitis may be seen in the form of endophthalmitis or pan-ophthalmitis and these are usually not shown in the exam setting.

Chronic non-suppurative choroidoretinitis is characterized by diminished vision and/or flashes of light. There is usually no redness or photophobia. Patches of round cell infiltration of the choroid may be seen as poorly defined white or yellowish areas. White patches are usually lined by black dense pigment. Since conditions like TB, toxoplasmosis and sarcoidosis may result in choroidoretinitis, systemic examination (enlargement of liver, lymph nodes, etc.) may be necessary to find the underlying cause for the choroidoretinitis.

CASE 69 RETINITIS PIGMENTOSA

Examiner

Examine this patient's fundi.

- Note the exudates as described for choroidoretinitis. They will be extensive and bilateral, with bone spicule appearance with areas of pigmentary clumps. The arterioles will be narrowed. The essential difference is that the exudates in retinitis pigmentosa interrupt the vessels since the exudates are much more superficial.
- Test visual acuity (impaired or blind).
- Look for any evidence of secondary optic atrophy.
- Check the visual fields (constriction of visual fields may be present).
- Request permission from examiner to test for motor and sensory neuropathy and ataxia since the presence of such features would point towards the diagnosis of Refsum's disease. Retinitis pigmentosa may also be seen in patients with the Laurence–Moon–Beidl syndrome (see Case 20).

Candidate

This patient has exudates in both eyes suggestive of retinitis pigmentosa. (The presence of ataxia and sensory and motor neuropathy indicates that the patient may have Refsum's disease.)

Examiner

Name three illnesses that are associated with retinitis pigmentosa.

Candidate

1. Refsum's disease.
2. Abetalipoproteinaemia.
3. Laurence–Moon–Beidl syndrome.

Examiner

What is Refsum's disease?

Candidate

Refsum's disease is characterized by peripheral neuropathy, cerebellar ataxia, and elevated cerebrospinal fluid protein without the presence of pleocytosis, deafness and ichthyosis. The condition is inherited as an autosomal recessive trait. Biochemically there is a defective metabolism of phytanic acid that becomes deposited in different tissues of the body including the eyes. There is no satisfactory treatment available. Phytanic acid-free diet and plasma exchange may help in preventing the progression of disease.

Discussion on retinitis pigmentosa

The clinical features of retinitis pigmentosa may vary but night blindness and constriction of visual fields usually occur. Rods are more affected than cones. The age of onset, inheritance pattern, and progress of disease may all vary. The condition is inherited as an autosomal recessive trait (ask for a family history) in approximately 40% of cases, autosomal dominant in 20% and sex-linked recessive in approximately 5% of cases. Between 30–40% of patients may have no family history and the mutation may be spontaneous. Fundoscopic examination reveals narrowed retinal arterioles and bone spicule appearance and areas of small irregular pigment clumps.

The progression of pigmentary changes often results in scotomas in the visual field; increasing visual field constriction causes progressive visual field impairment. Pallor of the disc and atrophy of the macula are common. Patients may also develop open angle glaucoma, posterior subcapsular cataract, myopia and vitreous detachment. There is no effective therapy for retinitis pigmentosa.

CASE 70 CENTRAL RETINAL ARTERY OCCLUSION (EMBOLISM)

Examiner

Examine this patient's fundi.

- A whitish, pale oedematous retina.
- Look at the macular area for the peculiar round 'cherry red' spot (bright red spot on the fovea).
- Note that the narrowed arterioles are attenuated and there may be streaky haemorrhages around the vessels.
- The retinal veins are narrowed and oligaemic.
- The optic disc may be pale and atrophied (see Case 65).
- Do not forget to check visual acuity (vision is completely lost as a result of sudden complete blindness in the affected eye).

Candidate

This patient has total loss of visual acuity (blind) in the right eye with features suggestive of central retinal artery occlusion (go on to list your findings).

Examiner

What are the common causes of the occlusion?

Candidate

The occlusion may result from an embolus arising from the heart (atrial fibrillation, infective endocarditis, atrial myxoma) or in the carotid artery (atheromatous plaque). Retinal artery itself may be involved as a part of the systemic illness in conditions like giant cell arteritis, polyarteritis nodosa, systemic lupus erythematosus, scleroderma or mixed connective tissue disease. Rarely, the retinal artery occlusion may also result from the raised intracranial pressure as seen in glaucoma.

Examiner

What is amaurosis fugax?

Candidate

Amaurosis fugax is said to exist when there is sudden and transient loss of vision in one eye. The entire field of vision may be lost. Conditions that may cause amaurosis fugax include thromboembolism (carotid artery stenosis, polycythaemia rubra vera, sickle cell disease), cardiac arrhythmias and collagen vascular disease.

Discussion on central retinal artery occlusion

Retinal artery occlusion may affect the central retinal artery or one of its branches. The onset of loss of vision is usually sudden and acute. The occlusion may result from several causes listed above. The fundoscopic findings in central retinal artery occlusion include a whitish and oedematous retina and the appearance of a characteristic cherry red spot at the macula. Marked narrowing of the arterioles with segmentation of the blood column may be seen both in the arterioles as well as the venules.

Occasionally some patients develop rubeosis iridis and glaucoma. In patients with occlusion of a branch of the central retinal artery, the fundoscopic examination will show the findings to be limited to the area of the fundus supplied by the branch of the retinal artery. Over a period of months to years the recanalization of the obstructive vessels may result in few residual signs in the retina.

CASE 71 RETINAL VEIN THROMBOSIS

Examiner

Examine this patient's eyes.

In the affected eye:

- Note diminished visual acuity and loss of visual fields.
- Striking feature is gross venous distension and numerous haemorrhages.
- Papilloedema and oedema of the rest of the retina is present.
- Microaneurysms and collateral vessels may be present.
- Look for exudates.

Candidate

The patient has features of retinal vein thrombosis in the left eye (list them. If you are not sure of the diagnosis just give your findings and hope that the examiner can drag it out of you.)

Examiner

How do you distinguish this condition from papilloedema?

Candidate

The visual acuity in papilloedema remains normal until the late stages whereas it is affected at an early stage in retinal vein thrombosis. Papilloedema is usually bilateral whereas retinal vein thrombosis is usually unilateral.

Examiner

What are the causes of retinal vein thrombosis?

Candidate

There are several conditions which predispose to retinal vein thrombosis:

1. Hyperviscosity syndrome (myeloproliferative disorders, myeloma).
2. Hypertension.
3. Diabetes mellitus.
4. Glaucoma and hypermetropia.

PART 7

Looking at the Hands

GENERAL ADVICE

Make up your mind on inspection where the pathology lies, i.e. is this rheumatology, neurology, dermatology, myopathy or another condition? This will enable you to quickly concentrate physical examination in that area.

Do not forget to ask the patient whether there is any pain in the hands before you touch them! If only one hand is painful then examine that one last and gently too. It might be easier for you to instruct the patient to move the joints actively first before you try passively.

Place both hands next to each other so that one is compared to the other. Getting the patient to outstretch them may bring out the clue to the diagnosis (e.g. wrist drop, tremor, ataxia).

Examine both the dorsal and the palmar aspects.

Joint swellings and deformities should be described according to position (distal interphalangeal joint, mid interphalangeal joint, proximal interphalangeal joint). Make sure the swelling is in the joint and not in the bone (bone cyst).

Go through the full range of joint movements for both hands and test power in all muscle groups.

When examining for nerve lesions do not forget to examine the wrist (traumatic or operative scar), neck (cervical rib/scar), eyelids (Horner's: T_1 lesion due to apical lung lesions leading to wasting of the first dorsal interosseus muscle), and face (acromegaly).

CASE 72 HANDS WITH JOINT SWELLINGS

Commonly given cases of joint swellings are:

a. Rheumatoid arthritis.
b. Psoriasis.
c. Osteoarthritis.
d. Gout.

Examiner

Examine this patient's hands.

Locally

- Note position of joint swelling or deformity (proximal interphalangeal joints are more commonly involved in rheumatoid arthritis. The distal interphalangeal joints are more commonly involved in osteoarthritis, psoriasis, gout and Reiter's syndrome).
- The patient may have both rheumatoid arthritis and osteoarthritis so look for presence of Heberden's nodes at the terminal interphalangeal joints.
- Look for Swan neck deformity or trigger finger (tendon sheath involvement) and Boutonnière (button hole) deformity.
- Examine for palmar erythema.
- Look for pitting of the nails to exclude psoriasis. Psoriatic arthropathy is seronegative and classically affects the terminal interphalangeal joints. No subcutaneous nodules are present in psoriasis.
- Lumpy swellings (tophi) around the joints sometimes with superficial ulceration and chalky material coming out of the shiny skin.
- Vasculitic lesions in the nail folds (rheumatoid arthritis) or pitting of the nails (psoriasis).
- Disuse of hands due to pain may result in muscle wasting which should be distinguished from ulnar and median nerve palsies.

Elsewhere look for

- Presence of subcutaneous nodules around the elbows should be looked for (present in rheumatoid arthritis, chronic gout).
- Tophi on the ear lobes.
- Psoriatic lesions on the skin especially the extensor aspects.
- Arthropathy of the other joints (knee, elbow, etc.)
- Nodules/scleromalacia of the eye.

Candidate

This patient has rheumatoid arthritis as evidenced by ... (give your physical findings).

Examiner

What two investigations may help the diagnosis?

1. X-ray of the hands (be prepared to list all the distinguishing features of rheumatoid arthritis from osteoarthritis).
2. Rheumatoid factor (latex or sheep red cell agglutination test).

Examiner

What is rheumatoid factor?

Candidate

These are IgG auto-antibiodies which react against self IgM or IgG antibodies.

Examiner

Name three pulmonary manifestations of rheumatoid arthritis.

Candidate

1. Diffuse pulmonary fibrosis.
2. Pleural effusion (exudate with low glucose and high LDH).
3. Pulmonary nodules.

Discussion on hands with joint swellings

Most cases of arthritis shown in the exam have long-standing changes of arthritis. In early rheumatoid arthritis, articular symptoms of rheumatoid arthritis and SLE may be similar. However, other clinical features (involvement of skin, lungs, heart, kidney, and blood changes) and laboratory investigations, etc. are helpful in differential diagnosis. The joint involvement in rheumatoid arthritis is usually bilateral and symmetrical and is most marked in the metacarpophalangeal (MCP) and proximal interphalangeal joints. The terminal interphalangeal joints are rarely involved. Ulnar deviation of the fingers at the MCP joints is common in rheumatoid arthritis.

In SLE similar changes may occur and this is called Jaccoud's arthropathy. Wrist joints are always affected. Swelling and limitation of the affected joints occurs and muscle wasting results as a consequence. Some patients with rheumatoid arthritis develop the carpal tunnel syndrome due to compression of the median nerve by the thickened and inflamed synovium. In hands severely affected by rheumatoid changes, the examiner will want you to have assessed the functional aspects of the hand, i.e. what can the patient usefully do with it? Hold a cup or spoon, etc. Physiotherapy, occupational therapy and joint replacements may be part of the discussion.

In osteoarthritis it is important to be familiar with the two types of nodes (Heberden's and Bouchard's). Heberden's nodes are typically seen as bony enlargements at the terminal interphalangeal joints. Bouchard's nodes are similar in nature but are present at the proximal interphalangeal joints. The first carpo-metacarpal joint may also be involved in osteoarthritis.

In chronic gout tophaceous deposits may be seen around or in the joints and tendons.

In psoriasis the involvement of nails and skin by the disease helps in the diagnosis. Terminal interphalangeal joints are typically affected.

Seronegative arthritides typically affect the terminal interphalangeal joints (psoriasis, Reiter's syndrome, osteoarthritis, gout).

CASE 73 ATROPHY OF THE SMALL MUSCLES OF THE HAND

Examiner

Examine this patient's hands.

Locally

- Examine both hands.
- On inspection, the wasting of the small muscles of the hand (thenar and hypothenar) will be obvious.
- Go on to test motor power and function of various muscles supplied by the median and ulnar nerves in the hand (see Cases 85, 86 and 87).
- Test for any sensory deficit and fasciculations.
- Look carefully for any evidence of rheumatoid arthritis (Case 72).

Elsewhere

With the examiner's permission:

- Examine upper limb reflexes.
- Look behind the elbows for evidence of possible trauma to the ulnar nerve.
- Look for features of Horner's syndrome (ptosis, miosis, enophthalmos).
- Examine the neck for any operation scar, cervical ribs, etc.
- Look for pyramidal signs in the lower limbs.

Candidate

This patient has wasting of the small muscles of the hand/s affecting the ... group of muscles. Then go on to give all the relevant physical signs seen.

Examiner

What are the common causes of small muscle wasting?

Candidate

There are several causes of wasting of the small muscles of the hand. These are:

1. Rheumatoid arthritis.
2. Peripheral nerve lesions, e.g. median and ulnar nerve lesions.
3. Spinal cord or nerve root lesions.
   a. Intramedullary (inside the spinal cord) e.g. motor neurone disease; syringomyelia; tumours.
   b. Extramedullary (outside the spinal cord) e.g. cervical spondylosis; cervical rib; tumours; apical lung tumours affecting T_1 root.

Examiner

What three investigations would you perform for a suspected myopathy?

Candidate

1. Serum creatine phosphokinase (CPK) estimation (typically raised in myopathy).
2. Electromyography (shows low amplitude contractions).
3. Muscle biopsy.

Examiner

What are the main differences between a myopathy and neuropathy?

Candidate

Go through the list in the Table below.

Differences between a myopathy and neuropathy

	Myopathy	*Neuropathy*
Muscular atrophy	Yes	Yes
Weakness	Usually proximal	Usually distal
Fasciculations	Absent	May be present
Sensory deficit	Absent	Present
Muscle enzymes	Raised	Normal
Diagnosis	Electromyography Muscle biopsy	Nerve conduction studies Nerve biopsy

Discussion on atrophy of the small muscles of the hand

There are many causes of small muscle atrophy of the hands that may or may not be symmetrical in both hands.

In **motor neurone disease** the reflexes in the upper limbs are usually brisk and not lost unless the muscles are grossly paralysed. Fasciculation is common and there is no sensory loss.

In **amyotrophic lateral sclerosis** pyramidal signs are present in the lower limbs.

In **syringomyelia** besides wasting there is patchy loss of pain and temperature sensation in both arms and sometimes there may be signs of Horner's syndrome on either side.

Spinal cord tumours are characterized by wasting, sensory disturbance and absent tendon reflexes in the upper limbs.

With Pancoast tumour of the lung and cervical rib, sensory loss in the ulnar nerve distribution commonly accompanies wasting of the small muscles.

Carpal tunnel syndrome, median and ulnar nerve lesions are discussed elsewhere (see Cases 83, 84, 87).

CASE 74 PALMAR ERYTHEMA

Examiner

Look at the hands and perform the relevant physical examination.

Locally

- Note the redness of the palms, especially over the thenar and hypothenar eminences and the pulps of the fingers.
- Exclude the presence of rheumatoid arthritis.

Elsewhere

- Since the most common association of palmar erythema is with liver disease, look for the following signs:

    - Dupuytren's contracture.
    - Spider naevi.
    - Leuconychia.
    - Jaundice.
    - Pallor.
    - Parotid gland enlargement.
    - Hepatosplenomegaly.
    - Ascites.
    - Leg oedema.
    - Gynaecomastia.
    - Absent secondary sexual hair.

- Rarely, the soles of the feet may also show redness.

Candidate

The hands show palmar erythema with presence/absence of signs of liver disease (list them if present).

Examiner

What are the common causes of palmar erythema?

Candidate

Palmar erythema is found in several conditions, namely:

1. Cirrhosis of the liver.
2. Pregnancy.
3. Females on contraceptive pills.
4. Thyrotoxicosis.
5. Rheumatoid arthritis.

Examiner

Name two conditions of the liver that predispose to an increased risk of hepatocellular carcinoma.

Candidate

1. Haemochromatosis.
2. Hepatitis B or hepatitis C.

Examiner

What is the role of serum ammonia estimation in liver disease?

Candidate

Serum ammonia estimation is an important test for monitoring the progress of hepatic encephalopathy. Although the ammonia level does not strictly correlate with encephalopathy, a falling serum ammonia level is usually associated with an improved clinical picture. The diagnosis of hepatic encephalopathy must be based on the total clinical picture of liver cell failure and, as such, measurement of blood ammonia level adds little to the clinical picture. Serum ammonia levels may also be high in other conditions including gastrointestinal bleeding, renal failure or even with high protein intake.

Discussion on palmar erythema

Palmar erythema is a persistent extensive redness of the palms of the hands due to local vasodilatation with increased blood flow. The cardiac output is usually increased in patients with prominent palmar erythema. Skin over the thenar, hypothenar and finger pulp eminences is markedly red compared to the rest of the palm. Some healthy adults may have some degree of palmar erythema.

CASE 75 DUPUYTREN'S CONTRACTURE

Examiner

Examine this patient's hands.

Locally

- Ask the patient to spread the fingers and look very carefully so that you do not miss this condition. The flexion deformity at the MCP joint of the ring and middle fingers will be obvious.
- Also make sure you examine both hands. The condition may be limited to one hand or may affect both hands. Early Dupuytren's contracture may be easily missed and it is better felt than seen. So palpate the palmar fascia.
- Look for palmar erythema, clubbing and leuconychia.
- Look for rheumatoid arthritis.

Elsewhere

- Since the most common association is cirrhosis of the liver look for signs mentioned in Case 74.
- Note that approximately 25% of patients with alcoholic liver cirrhosis have Dupuytren's contracture and painless parotid enlargement.

Candidate

This patient has Dupuytren's contracture of the left hand/right hand/both hands with/without signs of liver cirrhosis (list them if present).

Examiner

List four conditions which may cause Dupytren's contracture.

Candidate

1. Liver cirrhosis.
2. Rheumatoid arthritis.
3. Trauma (vibrating tools, gardeners).
4. May be familial.

Examiner

Name three factors which may contribute to ascites in cirrhosis.

Candidate

1. Portal hypertension.
2. Hypoproteinaemia.
3. Secondary hyperaldosteronism.

Examiner

Can you give four causes of anaemia in cirrhosis?

Candidate

1. Nutritional deficiency: most commonly folate and pyridoxine deficiency.
2. Blood loss due to peptic ulcer or oesophageal varices bleeding.
3. Hypersplenism/bone marrow depression.
4. Haemolysis.

Discussion on Dupuytren's contracture

The fibrosis and thickening of the palmar fascia and of the flexor tendons is the underlying pathology of Dupuytren's contracture. This subsequently results in the flexion deformity of the metacarpophalangeal joints, especially of the ring and the middle fingers and loss of function of the fingers. It is important to palpate the palms so that you do not miss the thickened fascia in patients with early Dupuytren's contracture.

In most cases the condition becomes bilateral. Dupuytren's contracture must be distinguished from ulnar nerve palsy which is characterized by the loss of function of the dorsal and palmar interossei muscles (loss of flexion of proximal phalanx, extension of dorsal phalanx, adduction and abduction of fingers). Loss of sensation over the ulnar border of the hand is also a feature of ulnar nerve palsy (see Case 85).

CASE 76 CLUBBING OF THE FINGERS

Examiner

Look at the hands and complete your examination appropriately.

Locally

- You are expected not only to recognize clubbing but also to come up with the most likely cause of clubbing in the given patient.
- Make sure there is clubbing:

  - Drumstick appearance of the finger terminus.
  - Thickened tissue at base of nail.
  - Loss of angle between the base of the nail and adjacent skin of finger.
  - Note the convexity of the nail from above, down as well as from side to side.
  - Be seen to examine for abnormal fluctuation at the nail bases.

- Look for splinter haemorrhages.
- Check for evidence of hypertrophic pulmonary osteo-arthropathy and painful swelling of the ends of the radius and ulna due to periosteal thickening.
- Look for wasting of the first dorsal interosseus muscle.

Elsewhere

- Look for dyspnoea and cyanosis.
- Examine chest for conditions such as bronchiectasis, lung abscess, carcinoma and fibrosing alveolitis.
- Examine the cardiovascular system for any evidence of congenital heart disease.

Candidate

This patient has clubbing of the fingers most likely due to (state what you think the likely cause in the patient is and why you think so).

What are the causes of clubbing?

Recognized causes of clubbing are:

1. Respiratory system:
   a. Bronchiectasis.
   b. Lung abscess.
   c. Carcinoma of lung.
   d. Fibrosing alveolitis.
2. Cardiovascular system:
   a. Cyanotic heart disease.
   b. Infective endocarditis.
   c. Atrial myxoma.
3. Liver and gastrointestinal tract:
   a. Crohn's disease.
   b. Ulcerative colitis.
   c. Coeliac disease.
   d. Primary biliary cirrhosis of the liver.
4. Familial/idiopathic clubbing.
5. Thyrotoxicosis (thyroid acropachy).

The exact pathogenesis of clubbing is unknown. Altered neurocirculatory reflexes leading to increased blood flow and tissue hypertrophy is thought to be the underlying mechanism (clubbing has been known to respond to vagotomy).

Discussion on clubbing of the fingers

Clubbing of the fingers is an important physical sign and may be the first indication of a serious underlying disease. Clubbing of the toes may also occur but is more difficult to recognize because the toes are bulbous. The features of clubbing are listed above. In the membership examination, the presence of clubbing in the short case should alert you to examining the patient for signs of respiratory, cardiovascular, thyroid and gut disease (listed above).

The examiner will usually give you a clue as to the system you must examine, e.g. when asked to examine the patient's respiratory system you will quickly identify clubbing. This will alert you to one of the four common respiratory causes of clubbing (lung abscess, bronchiectasis, fibrosing alveolitis, carcinoma). It is important to note that patients with chronic bronchitis, tuberculosis, emphysema, and bronchial asthma are not expected to have clubbing unless complicated by suppurative infection or bronchial carcinoma.

CASE 77 SPLINTER HAEMORRHAGES

Examiner

Look at this patient's fingernails (or)
Examine this patient's hands.

Locally

- Look very carefully when screening the nails so as not to miss these lesions.
- Look at fingernails of both hands.
- Look at the direction of the splinter haemorrhage (longitudinal or transverse).
- Request to look at the toe nails as well.

Elsewhere

Once you are certain of the presence of splinter haemorrhages, with the permission of the examiner, look for other features of infective endocarditis (heart murmurs, petechial haemorrhages in the conjunctival or oral mucosa, anaemia, splenomegaly, Osler's nodes, Roth spots, Janeway lesions, etc). Osler's nodes are small, tender and erythematous lesions most commonly seen in the pads of the fingers or the palms. Janeway lesions are raised haemorrhagic areas in the palms of the hands.

Candidate

This patient has longitudinal splinter haemorrhages in the nail beds of the fingers on the right hand (or wherever they are). There are no other obvious signs of infective endocarditis (or list them if there are).

Examiner

What common conditions are associated with splinter haemorrhages?

Candidate

There are several conditions which cause splinter haemorrhages:

1. Trauma.
2. Infective endocarditis.
3. Septicaemia.
4. Malignancy.
5. Scurvy.
6. Trichiniasis.

Examiner

What four investigations may be helpful in a patient with suspected infective endocarditis?

Candidate

1. Blood cultures.
2. Echocardiography.
3. ESR (usually over 80 mm).
4. Urinalysis (proteinuria, microscopic haematuria).

Examiner

Give three complications of infective endocarditis.

Candidate

1. Thromboembolism (stroke, mycotic aneurysm in the brain, splenic abscess).
2. Intractable heart failure.
3. Rupture of the papillary muscle.

Discussion on splinter haemorrhages

Nail bed haemorrhages usually have a linear longitudinal distribution near the distal end hence the term 'splinter' haemorrhages. Involvement of the fingers may vary and a single nail bed may have several areas of 'splinters'. Remember that these haemorrhages are not considered to be pathognomonic of infective endocarditis. Rarely, the toes may also be involved. Splinter haemorrhages occur due to trauma to capillaries or due to dissemination of tiny emboli. Trichiniasis (rare in the UK) causes transverse haemorrhages typically affecting all the nail beds simultaneously. The presence of splinter haemorrhages in a patient with fever and cardiac murmurs must arouse suspicion of infective endocarditis.

CASE 78 LEUCONYCHIA

Examiner

Look at the patient's nails.

Locally

- Look carefully at the nails of both hands. The whiteness of the whole nail or bands or flecks of whiteness (leuconychia) will be apparent.

Elsewhere

- Look for stigmata of liver cirrhosis (Case 44) and nephrotic syndrome.

Candidate

This patient has leuconychia and has signs of liver cirrhosis (list them) (or) of nephrotic syndrome (or) the patient has leuconychia but there are no obvious signs of liver disease or nephrotic syndrome. Other causes of leuconychia will have to be ruled out.

Examiner

What two investigations would you ask for?

Candidate

1. Liver function tests.
2. Urine examination (for proteinuria).

Discussion on leuconychia

Hypoalbuminaemia due to any cause may result in leuconychia. Thus cirrhosis of the liver, nephrotic syndrome, protein losing enteropathy and chronic inorganic arsenic poisoning are important causes. Do remember that small isolated white patches may sometimes be seen in the nails of normal persons. The white discoloration of the nail may occur in punctate or diffuse fashion. The whiteness of the nail may also appear in the form of transverse lines (Mee's lines). These lines are most commonly seen as a result of arsenic poisoning or infections. Local trauma to the nail is the most common cause for punctate leuconychia. Excessive whiteness of the nails may also be seen in other systemic conditions such as congestive cardiac failure, pulmonary tuberculosis, diabetes mellitus, rheumatoid arthritis and carcinomatosis.

CASE 79 MARFAN'S SYNDROME

Examiner

Look at the patient's hands and go on to perform the relevant examination.

Locally

- The long fingers will be immediately apparent (arachnoid-actaly).
- Examine for hyperextensibility of the fingers.

Elsewhere

- Look at the palate (high arched).
- Examine the eyes for subluxation of the lens and iridodenesis (abnormal tremulousness of the iris).
- Measure the patient's height and arm span (tall patient with an arm span greater than his height).
- Measure floor to pubis and pubis to crown height (floor to pubis height is more than pubis to crown height).
- Check for hyperextensibility of joints, flat feet and kypho-scoliosis.
- Listen for aortic or mitral regurgitation murmurs.

Candidate

This patient has Marfan's syndrome with the following characteristics. He has arachnoidactyly, hyperextensile joints, a high arched palate, subluxed eye lens, is tall with the arm span greater than his height, and has mitral regurgitation.

Examiner

Give three endocrine causes of a tall stature.

Candidate

1. Gigantism/acromegaly.

2. Hyperthyroidism.
3. Congenital adrenal virilizing tumour.

Examiner

How do you determine if a particular child has a tall stature?

Candidate

Tall stature is considered to be present if a child has a height greater than the 97th percentile as compared to the height of the normal population of the same age group. From the various graphs and tables one can find out the exact percentile of a child of any age group.

Discussion on Marfan's syndrome

Marfan's syndrome is an inherited connective tissue disorder of unknown aetiology. It is transmitted as an autosomal dominant trait. The clinical features include skeletal (tall stature, pectus deformities, arachnoidactyly, scoliosis), cardiovascular (aortic and mitral valve regurgitation, aortic aneurysm, and aortic dissection) and ocular abnormalities (lens dislocation and myopia). The disorder affects approximately 1 in 15 000 individuals with men and women being affected equally. There is a wide variability in clinical severity with members of the same family having different extents of involvement. Lens dislocation may result in cataract formation and glaucoma. Mitral valve prolapse is commonly present and mitral regurgitation develops in over 70% of cases.

Homocystinuria is an important differential diagnosis. This is an autosomal recessive disorder with clinical features resembling Marfan's syndrome and includes peripheral vascular disease, arterial thrombosis, lens dislocation and osteoporosis with increased tendency to bone fractures and mental retardation. The diagnosis is established by the presence of excessive homocystine in the urine. The presence of mitral valve prolapse alone, in the absence of other clinical features, should not be confused with Marfan's. Tall stature is also a feature of Klinefelter's syndrome (see Case 8). There is no satisfactory treatment of Marfan's syndrome. Patients should ideally be followed every year for ocular and cardiac (including echocardiographic) evaluation.

CASE 80 SYRINGOMYELIA/SYRINGOBULBIA

Examiner

Examine this patient's hands neurologically (or)
Examine this patient's hands.

Locally

- Note the wasting of the small muscles of the hands with or without trophic lesions.
- Check for segmental areas of loss of pain and temperature sensation and see if there is any scar of painless burn or cut on the fingers.
- Look for fasciculations.

Elsewhere (with the examiner's permission)

- Examine for signs of lower motor neurone lesions in the upper limbs (due to involvement of the anterior horn cells) and upper motor neurone lesions in the lower limbs (due to involvement of the pyramidal tracts).
- Look for signs of Horner's syndrome on either side (see Case 59). Look for presence of nystagmus (probably due to involvement of fibres of the vestibulospinal tracts).
- Look for fasciculations in upper limb muscles.

Candidate

This patient has syringomyelia as evidenced by (give your physical signs). If you are not sure of the diagnosis just spell out the physical signs.

Examiner

Name three investigations which may help you make the diagnosis.

Candidate

1. Myelogram.
2. CT scan.
3. Magnetic resonance imaging.

Examiner

List four differential diagnoses.

Candidate

1. Spinal cord tumour.
2. Motor neurone disease.
3. Multiple sclerosis.
4. Tabes dorsalis.

Discussion on syringomyelia/syringobulbia

Syringomyelia is a condition characterized by the presence of a cavity in the spinal cord (most commonly in the cervical region). If the cavity is present in the brainstem, the term syringobulbia is applied. In most cases the symptoms appear between the ages of 25 to 35 years and included sensory impairment and weakness and wasting of the hands. Patients may have an unsteady gait with progressive stiffness. Light touch sensation is preserved but pain and temperature sensation are lost.

Horner's syndrome may develop because of involvement of sympathetic fibres at C_8–T_1 level. The course of the disease is unpredictable. Some patients may have limited neurological deficit and continue to function well for many years after the diagnosis. In others, the disease may progress rapidly. There is no satisfactory treatment available. Surgical procedures include compression of the cavity or grafting of the muscle tissue.

CASE 81 HEBERDEN'S NODES

Examiner

Look at this patient's hands and tell me what your diagnosis is.

Locally

- Identify the swellings at the distal interphalangeal joints. Heberden's nodes are the osteophytes causing this swelling.
- Look for similar bony swellings at the proximal interphalangeal joints (Bouchard's nodes) and the metacarpophalangeal joints especially the first (thumb) metacarpophalangeal joint.
- Note that the patient is usually obese and elderly.

Elsewhere (with the examiner's permission)

- Look for evidence of osteoarthritis in other joints, especially the knees and hips.

Candidate

This patient has osteoarthritis as seen by . . . (list your findings).

Examiner

What single investigation would you ask for?

Candidate

X-ray of the hands.

Examiner

Name four radiological changes of osteoarthritis.

Candidate

1. Sclerosis of bone.
2. Narrowing of joint space.

3. New bone formation (osteophytes).
4. Alteration in the shape of the bony ends as seen in the head of the femur in osteoarthritis of the hip.

Discussion on Heberden's nodes

Heberden's nodes and Bouchard's nodes give the diagnosis away. In the early stages there is an element of inflammation that may cause pain and discomfort. With chronicity, the Heberden's nodes are visible as prominent nodes with angular deformities (flexion and lateral deviation of distal phalanges). These nodes are more commonly seen in women than in men (10:1). There is some evidence that the Heberden's nodes have some degree of hereditary tendency. The actual mode of transmission is not known. A single autosomal gene, dominant in females and recessive in males, has been suggested. Heberden's nodes are usually seen in the hands and not in the feet. The presence of Heberden's nodes has no direct correlation with the involvement of other joints by osteoarthritis.

CASE 82 SWELLING OF THE PHALANGES
(BONY CYSTS)

Examiner

Examine this patient's hands.

Locally

• Place both hands together with fingers wide apart.
• Once the swelling is identified, determine whether the swelling is in the joint, the soft tissue, or bone. Palpate the swelling and move the finger joint.
• Look at all fingers for similar involvement.

Elsewhere

• Look at the face for any evidence of lupus pernio (a bluish discoloration on the nose, not uncommonly seen in sarcoidosis).
• Examine the eyes (with permission) for uveitis.

Candidate

This patient has a bony swelling most likely to be a bony cyst. The presence of lupus pernio makes the likely diagnosis sarcoidosis.

Examiner

What two investigations may help the diagnosis?

Candidate

1. X-ray of the hands.
2. Serum angiotensin converting enzyme (SACE).
3. Kveim test.
4. Gallium scan.

What is Heerfordt's syndrome?

Heerfordt's syndrome is considered to be a variant of acute sarcoidosis and is characterized by the presence of:

1. Uveitis.
2. Facial nerve palsy.
3. Parotitis.

What are the common causes of swelling of the phalanges?

1. Sarcoidosis (bony cyst).
2. Sickle cell disease.
3. Chronic infection.

Discussion on swelling of the phalanges

Bone involvement in sarcoidosis is more common in black than white people. Most patients with bone involvement also have skin involvement. The metacarpals and terminal phalanges are most commonly affected. It is important to differentiate the involvement of the joints from the bone involvement. Joint involvement, seen in up to 40% of patients with acute sarcoidosis, may be in the form of monoarthritis or polyarthritis. Almost all joints, including ankles, knees, wrists and smaller joints of the hands, may be involved.

Most patients with joint involvement often have co-existing manifestations of erythema nodosum and hilar lymphadenopathy. Arthritis usually responds well to non-steroidal anti-inflammatory agents without any residual deformities. Bone pain and swelling are common features of bone infarction that may result from veno-occlusive crisis in sickle cell disease.

Bone infarction may also affect other joints and organs, especially the kidneys. Chronic non-healing skin ulcers are commonly present in these patients. Haemoglobin electrophoresis is helpful in confirming the diagnosis of sickle cell anaemia.

CASE 83 CARPAL TUNNEL SYNDROME

Examiner

This patient complains of a tingling sensation in his hands. Examine his/her hands.

Locally

- Examine the hands neurologically with a view to defining the neurological disorder and trying to identify the cause for it.
- Note that the neurological symptoms in the hand may be due to nerve lesions or compression at the wrist, forearm, arm or neck.
- Look for any scar of injury or bony deformity that might suggest previous trauma/operation to the wrist joint.
- Inspect for wasting of the small muscles of the hand, not forgetting the outer part of the thenar eminence. If present, then testing the muscles of the thumb, e.g. opponens and abductor pollicis brevis (supplied by the median nerve) for muscle power (weakness) is essential.
- Examine for sensory loss (in carpal tunnel syndrome there will be loss/diminished sensation over the palmar aspects of the thumb, index finger, middle and radial half of the ring fingers – sensation over the rest of the palm is normal).
- Look for features of rheumatoid arthritis.
- Percuss over the carpal ligament and ask the patient whether he experiences paraesthesiae (Tinel's sign).
- Check for Phalen's sign (see discussion section, below).

Elsewhere

- Look for features of acromegaly, hypothyroidism and amyloidosis.

Candidate

This patient has the carpal tunnel syndrome as evidenced by . . . (list signs and give the most likely cause if you have identified it).

Examiner

What are the common causes of this syndrome?

Candidate

1. Local trauma.
2. Rheumatoid arthritis.
3. Acromegaly.
4. Hypothyroidism.
5. Pregnancy.
6. Premenstrual oedema.

Examiner

Name three occupations that are commonly associated with carpal tunnel syndrome.

Candidate

1. Carpenters.
2. Painters.
3. Power saw/drill operators.

Discussion on carpal tunnel syndrome

Carpal tunnel syndrome develops as a result of the compression of the median nerve between the tendons of the hand muscles and the transverse carpal ligament in the volar aspect of the wrist. The most common clinical findings, apart from the median nerve compression signs, are the positive Tinel's test and the Phalen's sign. In Tinel's sign the pain and paraesthesiae are felt in the area of the median nerve distribution upon tapping over the area of the median nerve at the flexor aspect of the wrist. In Phalen's sign the pain and/or paraesthesiae occurs when both hands are jointly maintained in the extreme flexion position for approximately one minute.

CASE 84 ABSENT RADIAL PULSE (EITHER SIDE)

This case is often used to ascertain whether the candidate has a systematic approach to examination of the pulses of both sides.

Examiner

Examine the peripheral vascular system (or)
Examine the cardiovascular system.

Locally

- Check both radial pulses simultaneously and assess the difference in volume of both right and left radial pulses.
- On the side where the radial pulse is absent or feeble go on to feel for the brachial, axillary and subclavian arteries respectively.
- Listen for any carotid/vertebral bruits on both sides of the neck.
- Look for any mass compressing the neck.

Candidate

This patient has a feeble volume/absent radial pulse on the left/right side ... (then proceed to give other findings).

Examiner

What is pulseless (Takayasu's) disease?

Candidate

It is a rare condition first described by Takayasu in Japan which is characterized by arteritis and occurs particularly in young women. All three major trunks arising from the aortic arch are affected resulting in coronary insufficiency, absent pulses in the arms, and symptoms of cerebral ischaemia.

Examiner

What is subclavian steal syndrome?

Candidate

It is a rare condition in which symptoms of vertebrobasilar insufficiency are experienced by the patient on exercising his arm since the subclavian artery distal to the stenosis steals blood retrogradely from the vertebral artery. The condition is seen in cases of subclavian artery stenosis at or near its origin.

Examiner

How is the circle of Willis in the brain formed?

Candidate

Anterior, posterior and middle cerebral arteries join through anterior and posterior communicating arteries to form the circle of Willis.

Discussion on absent radial pulse

Other common peripheral vascular conditions which appear in the short cases include:

1. Abnormal position of the radial artery.
2. Thrombosis/embolism in a peripheral (upper or lower limb) artery.
3. Takayasu's arteritis.
4. Subclavian artery stenosis.
5. Brachial artery catheter.
6. A–V shunt (for dialysis).
7. Deep vein thrombosis.

CASE 85 CLAW HANDS (ULNAR NERVE PALSY)

Examiner

Examine this patient's hand(s).

Locally

- Always examine both hands.
- The claw hand/s will be immediately apparent. Note that the proximal (MCP joint) phalanges are overextended and the interphalangeal joints are flexed, with slight separation of the ring and little fingers. Wasting of small muscles is present.
- Test all muscle groups of the hand and forearm.
- Test for sensory loss. Ulnar nerve lesions cause loss of sensation in the T_1/C_8 distribution, i.e. ulnar border of the hand both on the dorsal and palmar aspects of the hand, the little finger and the ulnar half of the ring finger.
- If both hands are affected, the lesion is likely to be more central, i.e. at C_8/T_1 level.

Elsewhere

- Look around the olecranon groove and wrist for any visible scar or fracture as evidence of possible injury to the ulnar nerve.

Candidate

This patient has a right claw hand with signs of right ulnar nerve palsy (go on to describe them and give any other physical findings).

Examiner

What are the likely causes of bilateral claw hands with ulnar nerve palsies?

Candidate

More central lesions affecting the cord are more likely. Examples are: syringomyelia, motor neurone disease, cervical spondylosis and cervical cord tumours. In developing countries leprosy may be a common cause.

What are the two commonest causes of peripheral ulnar nerve lesions in the world?

1. Trauma.
2. Leprosy.

Brief me on the various cord segments, the upper limb muscles they supply and their action.

The cord segments C..T.. supply the muscles ... and whose action is tested by ... (go through Table below).

Cord segments	Muscles supplied	Action to be tested
$C_{7,8}$, T_1	Flexor carpi ulnaris	Ulnar flexion of hand
$C_{7,8}$, T_1	Flexor digitorum profundus (medial half)	Flexion of terminal phalanx of ring and little fingers against resistance
C_8, T_1	Adductor pollicis	Adduction of metacarpal of thumb, by asking patient to attempt to hold a piece of paper between the thumb and palmar aspect of the forefinger
C_8, T_1	Abductor digiti minimi	Abduction of little finger
$C_{7,8}$, T_1	Opponens digiti minimi	Opposition of little finger
$C_{7,8}$, T_1	Flexor digiti minimi	Flexion of little finger
C_8, T_1	Dorsal and palmar interossei and lumbricals III and IV	Flexion of proximal phalanx, extension of two distal phalanges, and adduction and abduction of fingers

CASE 86 WRIST DROP (RADIAL NERVE PALSY)

Examiner

Examine this patient's hands.

Locally

- The wrist drop will be apparent when you ask the patient to stretch out both hands.
- The patient is unable to extend the wrists, the fingers at the metcarpophalangeal joints, and the thumb of the affected hand.
- Test for sensation (affected areas will be the posterior aspect of the thumb and the dorsoradial side of the hand. If the nerve is damaged higher up, above the origin of the posterior cutaneous nerve, a strip along the posterior surface of the forearm may show a loss of sensation).

Elsewhere

- Look for any scar or injury especially in the spiral groove on the shaft of the humerus.

Candidate

This patient has a right/left radial nerve palsy. The features which suggest this diagnosis are ... (present them).

Examiner

What are the causes of a radial nerve palsy?

Candidate

Trauma to the radial nerve along its path:

1. Fractures of the shaft of the humerus particularly at the junction of the middle and distal thirds.
2. Elbow injuries.

3. Chronic lead poisoning.
4. Saturday night palsy resulting from bizarre sleeping posture.
5. Conditions causing polyneuropathy (see Case 87).

Discussion on wrist drop

Remember the cord segments, muscles supplied and their actions, as given below.

Cord segments	Muscles supplied	Action to be tested
C_{6-8}	Triceps and anconeus	Extension of forearm
$C_{5,6}$	Brachioradialis	Flexion of forearm
C_{5-7}	Extensor carpiradialis	Radial extension of hand
C_{6-8}	Extensor digitorum	Extension of phalanges of all four fingers in the hand
C_{6-8}	Extensor digiti minimi	Extension of phalanges of little finger
C_{6-8}	Extensor carpi ulnaris	Ulnar extension of hand
C_{5-7}	Supinator	Supination of forearm
$C_{6,7}$	Abductor pollicis longus	Abduction of metacarpal of thumb
$C_{6,7}$	Extensor pollicis brevis	Extension of thumb
C_{6-8}	Extensor digitorum longus	Extension of index finger

CASE 87 MEDIAN NERVE PALSY

Examiner

Examine this patient's hands neurologically.

Locally

- Look for any scar or injury around the wrist.
- Note the wasting of the thenar eminence, and the thumb falling into a flat ape-like position.
- Test for loss of sensation in the volar aspect of the thumb, index and middle fingers.
- Remember to test for muscle functions supplied by the median nerve as given below.

Cord segments	Muscles supplied	Action to be tested
$C_{6,7}$	Pronator teres	Pronation of forearm
$C_{6,7}$	Flexor carpi radialis	Radial flexion of hand
$C_{6,7}$ T_1	Palmaris longus	Flexion of hand
$C_{7,8,}$ T_1	Flexor digitorum superficialis	Flexion of middle phalanx of all four fingers
$C_{6,7}$	Flexor pollicis longus	Flexion of terminal phalanx of thumb
$C_{7,8,}$ T_1	Flexor digitorum profundus	Flexion of terminal phalanx of index and middle fingers
$C_{6,7}$	Abductor pollicis brevis	Abduction of metacarpal of thumb
$C_{6,7}$	Flexor pollicis brevis	Flexion of proximal phalanx of thumb
$C_{6,7}$	Opponens pollicis	Opposition of metacarpal of thumb
$C_{8,}$ T_1	Two lateral lumbricals	Flexion of proximal phalanx and extension of the two distal phalanges of index and middle fingers

Candidate

This patient has median nerve palsy as evidenced by (list your physical signs).

Examiner

What is mononeuritis multiplex?

Candidate

The term mononeuritis multiplex is used when there is a simultaneous or sequential involvement of multiple peripheral nerves. The motor and/or sensory deficit is limited to the distribution of the particular nerve. The peripheral nerves may be involved randomly and the degree of involvement may vary in different nerves. Common causes of mononeuritis multiplex include:

1. Rheumatoid arthritis.
2. Diabetes mellitus.
3. Polyarteritis nodosa.
4. Systemic lupus erythematosus.
5. Sarcoidosis.
6. Leprosy.
7. Amyloidosis.

Discussion on median nerve palsy

Learn some of the common causes of peripheral neuropathy. The list is exhaustive but some examples are listed:

1. Metabolic.

    – Diabetes. mellitus, porphyria, uraemia.

2. Vitamin deficiency.

    – B1, B2, B6 (commonly associated with alcoholism).
    – B12.

3. Toxic neuropathy.

   – Lead, arsenic, aniline dyes.

4. Drugs.

   – Dilantin, nitrofurantoin, vincristine, isoniazide, chloroquine, lithium, colchicine, hydralazine.

5. Trauma.
6. Infective.

   – Leprosy, Guillain Barré syndrome.

7. Miscellaneous.
   – Multiple myeloma, remote effects of malignancy (e.g.
   lung), hereditary neuropathies, snake bites.

CASE 88 INTENTION TREMOR

Examiner

Examine the hands/upper limbs neurologically.

Locally

- During your examination the intention tremor (ataxic movements which appear on intention and disappear at rest) will be obvious.
- Test both upper limbs for intention tremor asking the patient to perform a function.
- Look for other signs of cerebellar disease, e.g. finger to nose test for ataxia, scanning speech dysarthria, nystagmus, hypotonia, titubation.

Elsewhere

With the examiner's permission, look for upgoing plantar reflexes with spasticity of the lower limb (since patients with multiple sclerosis are common short cases).

Candidate

This patient has an intention tremor with signs of cerebellar disease (go on to list them).

Examiner

What types of tremor do you know?

Candidate

Common types of tremor are:

1. Tremor at rest.
2. Postural tremor.
3. Flapping tremor.
4. Senile tremor.

5. Essential familial tremor.
6. Hysterical tremor.

Discussion on intention tremor

Tremor is a rhythmical stereotyped movement of antagonistic groups of muscles. Features of the various types of tremors are:

1. **Tremor at rest**: this is characteristically seen in parkinsonism; these are present at rest and disappear on intention/action. The tremor may be described as a 'pill rolling' tremor because simultaneous movements of the fingers and thumbs in a pill-rolling fashion occur. The tremors worsen on emotional excitement but disappear during sleep. Other associated features of parkinsonism (rigidity, dyskinesia, festinating gait, etc.) are useful in diagnosing the condition (see Case 21).

2. **Postural tremor**: these tremors are also known as 'action tremors' since they are best seen on outstretched arms in conditions including anxiety, neurosis, thyrotoxicosis, alcoholism, and uraemia. Occasionally these tremors may also be present in healthy adults.

3. **Flapping tremors (asterixis)** these are seen in outstretched arms with hands dorsiflexed in patients with hepatic cell, respiratory failure or toxic states. Patients typically have other stigmata of liver disease (see Case 46 for other information).

4. **Intention tremor** the tremor becomes prominent as the limb approaches a target; the tremor disappears at rest. Intention tremors are characteristic of diseases of the cerebellum or its connection with the brainstem (extrapyramidal system).

5. **Senile tremor** these are seen with ageing. Tremors are fine and rapid (relatively slow and coarse in parkinsonism). These are present on intention or at rest. There is no associated rigidity or bradykinesia. No treatment is usually required.

6. **Essential familial tremor** (see Case 24).

7. **Hysterical tremor** these may be fine or coarse and may vary from time to time. Tremors are usually unilateral but may also be bilateral. Other associated features of hysteria are helpful in diagnosis.

PART 8

Looking at the Legs

GENERAL ADVICE

As with examination of the hands, examine both legs and place them together for comparison. Make sure that both legs are adequately exposed up to the groins.

Asking the patient to walk is an essential part of the examination and will reveal many physical signs. While the patient is standing, perform the Romberg's test.

Go through the inspection, palpation, movement and neurology routine (fasciculations, bulk, power, tone, reflexes/clonus, extrapyramidal signs).

Do not forget to examine the back of the legs and the vertebral column (Gibbus or operation scar).

CASE 89 PAGET'S DISEASE: BOWING OF THE LEGS

Examiner

Examine this patient's legs.

Locally

- The lateral bowing of the leg(s) will be obvious.
- Palpate and feel whether the local temperature of the affected area over the bone (on both sides) is raised. This may be increased due to increased vascularity and arterio-venous fistula.
- The subcutaneous surface of the tibia is often widened.
- Occasionally a bruit may be audible locally.
- Look for oedema of the legs (a feature of congestive cardiac failure which is associated with Paget's disease of the bone).

Elsewhere (with the examiner's permission)

- Look at the skull for enlarged calvarium since the skull is commonly affected.
- Look for deformities of the other bones if present, e.g. pelvis, humerus, spine, clavicle, etc.
- Look for signs of high output cardiac failure, e.g. collapsing pulse, raised JVP, cardiomegaly, hepatomegaly and oedema of legs as mentioned earlier.
- Check for deafness.

Candidate

This patient has Paget's disease of the bone as seen by ... (list your signs). Alternatively, say 'This patient has the following physical signs' and hope the examiner will ask you for a differential diagnosis.

Examiner

What are the common causes of bowed legs?

Candidate

Bowing of the legs may be a feature of:

1. Paget's disease of the bone.
2. Rickets or osteomalacia.
3. Sabre tibia (where bowing of the legs is anteriorly and is due to congenital syphilis).

Examiner

Discuss the differential diagnosis of the three causes of bowing of the legs you have listed.

Candidate

(Go through the Table on the next page).

Discussion on Paget's disease: bowing of the legs

Paget's disease of the bone is seldom seen before the age of 50 years and its aetiology remains unknown. There is evidence of both increased osteoblastic and osteoclastic activity. Both men and women are affected equally. The condition remains asymptomatic in over 70% of cases and the diagnosis may come to light only because of an incidental X-ray finding of Paget's disease of one or more bones (see Case 1).

Differentiating features of Paget's disease, osteomalacia and sabre tibia

Paget's disease	Rickets	Sabre tibia (congenital syphilis)
Patient is usually of normal height but with a stoop	Patient is usually of short stature	Patient is usually a dwarf
Skull commonly involved, with enlarged calvarium with an irregular surface. Also, deafness may be present due to 8th nerve involvement	Bossing of frontal and parietal bones	Bossing of frontal and parietal bones; a depressed bridge of nose due to 'snuffles' may be seen
Pelvis, humerus, clavicle, tibia and femur may be involved	Pelvic deformities may be seen. In the chest: 'rickety rosary', pigeon chest, funnel chest, Harrison's sulcus and kyphoscoliosis may be seen	Other stigmata of congenital syphilis, e.g. interstitial keratitis, corneal opacity, choroiditis, optic atrophy, Hutchinsons' incisors (notched and peg-shaped teeth) may be present
Bowing of the legs with rise in temperature over the legs due to increased vascularity	Bowing of both legs but no evidence of increased vascularity	Sabre tibia may be unilateral and the bowing is anteriorly and not laterally
There may be evidence of high output cardiac failure	No evidence of high output cardiac failure	No evidence of high output cardiac failure
Biochemical findings	(active rickets)	
Calcium – normal	– normal or low	– normal
Phosphorus – normal	– low	– normal
Alkaline phosphatase – raised	– raised	– normal

CASE 90 SWELLING OF ONE LEG

Examiner

Look at the patient's leg and then go on to examine him appropriately.

Locally

- Determine whether oedema is pitting or non-pitting.
- Compare skin colour with other leg.
- Determine whether the local temperature of the skin is raised.
- Request the examiner's permission and say that you would like to elicit a Homan's sign (forced dorsiflexion of the foot leading to discomfort in the upper calf – this test is non-specific, insensitive and may dislodge a thrombus).
- Measure the mid-calf circumference (from a measured reference point above the medial malleolus of both legs).
- Examine knee joint posteriorly (ruptured Baker's cyst).

Elsewhere

- Check for any lymphadenopathy in the groins.
- Look for any abdominal mass causing obstruction to the venous flow of the leg.
- Look for evidence of rheumatoid arthritis elsewhere.

Candidate

This patient has unilateral swelling of the left calf whose circumference is ... centimetres greater than the right (then go on to giving all your physical signs).

Examiner

What are your differential diagnoses?

Candidate

There are four differential diagnoses:

1. Deep vein thrombosis of the leg.
2. Cellulitis of the leg.
3. Lymphoedema.
4. Ruptured Baker's cyst.

Examiner

How would you confirm your diagnosis?

Candidate

Diagnosis of deep vein thrombosis is difficult on clinical grounds alone. The following tests will help make a diagnosis:

1. Venography.
2. Impedance plethysmography.
3. Radio-iodine-labelled fibrinogen leg scanning.
4. Ultrasound/arthrogram.
5. Lymphangiogram.

Discussion on swelling of one leg

Deep vein thrombosis of the deep leg veins is a common condition and always carries a risk of pulmonary embolism. Damage to the vessel wall, reduced blood flow and increased coagulability of the blood are important causes to be considered. The clinical features of venous thrombosis include leg pain, swelling, tenderness, and discouloration of the skin. The thrombosed vessel may also be palpable occasionally as a cord. The precise diagnosis of deep vein thrombosis may be difficult on clinical grounds alone. Objective testing by the tests listed above (1–4) may fail to demonstrate any evidence of thrombosis in 40–50% of patients complaining of significant leg pain and swelling. On the other hand, patients with less convincing features may turn out to have extensive deep vein thrombosis.

CASE 91 SWELLING OF BOTH LEGS
(OEDEMA/LYMPHOEDEMA)

Examiner

Examine this patient's legs.

Locally

- Determine whether the oedema is pitting (venous) or non-pitting (lymphatic), but do remember that if venous oedema is chronic enough, it may become non-pitting.
- Check temperature and colour of overlying skin.
- Look for infection between the toes.
- Look for varicose veins.
- Measure the girth of both legs.
- Look for lymphadenopathy in the groins.
- Remember that most patients are obese middle-aged females if the swelling is due to primary lymphoedema (Milroy's disease).

Elsewhere (with the examiner's permission)

Look for signs of cardiac failure; hypoalbuminaemia due to nephrotic syndrome or cirrhosis of the liver, especially if the oedema is bilateral and pitting. Cardiac failure: raised JVP, hepatomegaly, heart murmurs and basal crepitations in the lungs. With progressive cardiac failure the oedema may extend to the thighs or the scrotum. In bedridden patients sacral oedema may be present. Hypoalbuminaemia: look for renal enlargement; puffiness over the eyelids; stigmata of cirrhosis.

Candidate

This patient has bilateral, pitting venous oedema due to congestive cardiac failure. Alternatively, say: This patient has bilateral lymphatic oedema with no signs of cardiac or renal failure nor of cirrhosis of the liver. Given that the patient is obese and a middle-aged female, the diagnosis is most likely to be Milroy's disease or primary lymphoedema.

Examiner

Is there any question you would like to ask the patient?

Candidate

Because primary lymphoedema runs in families I would like to ask for a family history of the condition.

Examiner

What other conditions cause such lymphoedema?

Candidate

Four other conditions come to mind:

1. Filarial lymphoedema (elephantiasis).
2. Yellow nail syndrome.
3. Neoplastic infiltration of the lymph nodes.
4. Surgical excision of the lymph nodes.

Discussion on swelling of both legs

Primary lymphoedema (Milroy's disease) predominantly affects females: the onset of clinical features is before the age of 40 years in most cases. Milroy's disease is a form of primary lymphoedema that is inherited as an autosomal dominant trait. Filariasis (due to the filarial worms *Wuchereria bancrofti* and *Brugia malayi*) in its end stage causes lymphoedema of the legs and the genitalia. By the time chronic lymphoedema manifests, the disease is usually burnt out. A rare condition, commonly talked about in the MRCP exam, is the yellow nail syndrome which is characterized by poor nail growth, yellowing of the nails, and multiple lymphatic abnormalities that may cause recurrent pleural effusion and swelling of the legs due to lymphoedema.

CASE 92 GANGRENE OF THE TOES

Examiner

Look at the foot and proceed to the relevant physical examination.

Locally

- Note the area of black discolouration over the toe or part of the foot.
- The area proximal to the gangrene may show atrophic changes: pale, cold, and shiny with the presence of superficial ulcers.
- Palpate the peripheral arteries (dorsalis pedis; posterior tibial; popliteal and femoral) for arterial insufficiency both on the side of the gangrene and on the other leg.
- If the femoral and popliteal arteries are not palpable, auscultate for a bruit over that artery and listen to determine whether or not the pulsations are present.
- Examine the lower limb for any evidence of peripheral neuropathy, since in cases of diabetes mellitus the two conditions may co-exist.

Elsewhere (with the examiner's permission)

- Look for signs of diabetes mellitus (eye, skin, etc.).
- Look for evidence of nicotine staining of fingers.
- Look for signs of rheumatoid arthritis, SLE.

Candidate

This patient has gangrene of the toes with ... (give all other physical signs).

Examiner

What are the common causes of toe gangrene?

The common causes of gangrene of the toes are:

1. Atherosclerosis.
2. Arterial embolism.
3. Thromboangiitis obliterans (Buerger's disease).
4. Collagen vascular disease (SLE, polyarteritis nodosa, rheumatoid arthritis, etc.).

Examiner

What single investigation would you perform?

Candidate

Random/fasting blood sugar estimation.

Discussion on gangrene of the toes

Ischaemia occurring as a result of progressive atherosclerosis, is usually characterized by dryness, loss of nail changes, loss of hair, ulceration and inelasticity of the skin. With severe obliteration of the blood supply, the tissues may lose their viability and gangrene with black discolouration and necrosis may develop. Loss of pulsation of the peripheral arteries is common. More than 50% of patients are diabetic. Patients may also have evidence of generalized vascular disease including myocardial infarction, carotid artery stenosis and strokes. Sudden occlusion of a major artery may occur from thrombosis at site or embolism of plaques.

A diabetic patient may develop gangrene from trivial injury to the toe. In most cases with dry gangrene the gangrenous toe may fall off without any surgery. In infected or wet gangrene, the associated toxaemia requires the use of antibiotics and amputation at an early stage. Meningococcal septicaemia and other states causing disseminated intravascular coagulation (DIC) may result in shock with digital gangrene.

CASE 93 LEG ULCER

Examiner

Examine this patient's legs.

Locally

- Note the site, size, surface, and edges of the ulcer.
- Palpate the peripheral arteries for evidence of peripheral vascular disease.
- Look for varicose eczema, with or without varicose veins.

Elsewhere (with the examiner's permission)

- Hands: look for evidence of arthropathy.
- Face: look for xanthelasmata.
- Abdomen: splenomegaly.

Candidate

This patient has a leg ulcer situated on the medial malleolus. The features of the ulcer are . . . (go on to describe them and then give all other positive physical signs).

Examiner

What are the common causes of leg ulcers?

Candidate

Leg ulcers are seen with a number of conditions:

1. Peripheral vascular disease.
2. Rheumatoid arthritis.
3. Diabetes mellitus.
4. Varicose veins.
5. Trauma.
6. Sickle cell disease.
7. Syphilis.

8. Leishmaniasis.
9. Tuberculosis.

Discussion on leg ulcer

Several features of the ulcers or associated signs may help distinguish the aetiology of the ulcers:

1. Varicose ulcers

Varicose incompetency causing increasing oedema, eczema and secondary bacterial infection commonly results in varicose ulceration around the ankles – most commonly around internal malleolus, lower and medial aspect of the leg. Remember that the 'eczema' in varicose ulcers is due to brownish haemosiderin pigmentation and not due to eczematous skin rash.

2. Ischaemic ulcers

These are commonly seen in the extreme degree of peripheral vascular disease. The limb is usually cold to touch and with poor or absent peripheral pulses.

3. Rheumatoid arthritis

The ulcers are usually over the lower legs and tend to be deep and indolent. There may be areas of vasculitis in the finger tips. The presence of rheumatoid hands would also support the diagnosis.

4. Necrobiosis lipoidica diabeticorum

These lesions are yellowish red sclerotic plaques most commonly seen on shins with ulceration.

5. Pyoderma gangrenosum

The ulcers have elevated purulent borders with gross undermining of the skin and a zone of erythema beyond the edge. These ulcers are commonly seen on the legs but sometimes may involve the trunk. Besides ulcerative colitis, multiple myeloma and leukaemia are other conditions associated with these ulcers.

6. Sickle cell anaemia

Punched out, sharply marginated round or oval ulcers in a coloured patient should lead the candidate to suspect sickle cell disesase as a cause. Hereditary spherocytosis, thalassaemias, thrombotic thrombocytopenic purpura and polycythaemia rubra vera may also be associated with the leg ulcers.

7. Traumatic ulcers
In healthy individuals the ulcer heals satisfactorily. Infected ulcers, particularly in a diabetic, tend to heal slowly.

8. Syphilitic ulcer
Occasionally in cases of tertiary syphilis, a sloughing gummatous ulcer with punched out edges may be seen, most commonly below the knees.

9. Tuberculous ulcers
Chronic ulcers with undermined skin edges may involve an area of the leg. Lupus vulgaris (more common on the face, less commonly in the legs) is usually characterized by scaliness of the ulcer edges and scarring of the centre.

CASE 94 GOUT (BIG TOE)

Examiner

If there is a patient in the ward with acute gout it is almost certain that this patient will be shown as a short case (or a long case) for the MRCP.

Examiner

Examine the feet and tell me what the most likely diagnosis is.

Locally

• The red, tender swelling of the metatarsophalangeal joint will be obvious. The big toe is the first joint to be affected in 85% of cases.

Elsewhere

• Examine for swelling and deformity of other joints since the chronic form can become polyarticular.
• Look carefully for the presence of tophi which consist of deposits of urates in the periarticular tissues and the cartilages of the ears.
• Look for anaemia, bleeding gums.

Candidate

This patient's right big toe is swollen, tender and inflamed although no other joints are affected nor are there any tophi elsewhere. This patient has acute gouty arthritis.

Examiner

What three investigations would you request?

Candidate

1. Full blood count (polycythaemia, leukaemia).
2. Serum uric acid.
3. X-ray of the affected joint.

Examiner

What are three common precipitating factors for an acute gouty attack?

Candidate

1. Alcohol intake.
2. Thiazide diuretic.
3. Trauma.

Examiner

What are the three most useful drugs for an acute attack?

Candidate

1. Colchicine.
2. Indomethacin.
3. Phenylbutazone.

Examiner

What are the three differential diagnoses?

Candidate

1. Local cellulitis.
2. Simple trauma to the joint.
3. Pyogenic arthritis.

Discussion on gout

Acute gouty attack is characterized by an acute swelling of the joint, most commonly the metatarsophalangeal joint of the big toe. Other joints, including the ankle and the hands, may be involved. Although the serum uric acid may be normal, over 95% of patients have hyperuricaemia. Monosodium urate crystals are deposited in the joints and the tendons, because of supersaturation of body fluids; the acute inflammation of the joint results because of periarticular deposition of urate crystals. Under the polarizing microscope, the monosodium urate crystals are seen as negatively birefringent and are considered to be pathognomonic of the diagnosis.

The condition must be differentiated from pseudogout (chondrocalcinosis) which is characterized by the presence of positively birefringent crystals of calcium pyrophosphate. Chronic gout is characterized by hyperuricaemia and erosive arthropathy due to urate deposition in the joints, bursae and the tendons. In many cases the tophaceous deposits on the skin (hands, ears and feet) erupt and discharge chalky urate crystals. Urate stones may develop in the kidneys because of persisting high levels of urate in the blood and the urine.

CASE 95 ERYTHEMA NODOSUM

Examiner

Look at the patient's legs.

Locally

- Note the subcutaneous, rounded, tender nodules up to 5 cm in diameter on the anterior surface of the shins.

Elsewhere (with examiner's permission)

- Look for similar lesions on the extensor surface of the arms.
- Look into the throat for any evidence of tonsillitis or pharyngitis (although since this precedes EN by 2–3 weeks, the findings are often normal).
- Examine the respiratory system for any evidence of tuberculosis.
- Look for signs which will suggest sarcoidosis (lupus pernio, eye signs).

Candidate

This patient has lesions typical of erythema nodosum

Examiner

What are the common causes of erythema nodosum?

Candidate

1. Streptococcal infections.
2. Pregnancy.
3. Sarcoidosis.
4. Drug sensitivity (contraceptive pill, aspirin, sulphonamide).
5. Mycobacterial infections (e.g. TB/leprosy).
6. Fungal infections (e.g. histoplasmosis).

7. Chlamydial infections (e.g. psittacosis, LGV).
8. Rheumatic fever.
9. Idiopathic.

Examiner

What single question would you like to ask the patient?

Candidate

Have you taken any medication/drugs recently?

Examiner

What three investigations would you ask for?

Candidate

1. Chest X-ray.
2. ASO titres.
3. Mantoux test.

Other acceptable answers:

4. Kviem test/gallium scan/SACE levels.
5. Chlamydia serology, etc.

Discussion on erythema nodosum

Erythema nodosum is typically characterized by the presence of painful, subcutaneous, bilateral erythematous nodules over the pretibial areas. The lesions appear as dusky, red and tender nodules. The extensor surface of the upper limbs can also be involved. Women are affected more commonly than men (3:1). Fever and arthralgia (most commonly ankle joints) are common. There are several known causes (see list above), although in up to 50% of cases the cause may remain unknown. The condition is thought to be a hypersensitivity vasculitis (type III mediated immune complex).

Biopsy of the nodules reveals panniculitis affecting the subcutaneous connective tissues. In most cases patients recover between 4–6 weeks without any residual scarring or joint damage. Ecchymotic bruised appearance may last for several weeks. In some cases the skin lesions may be recurrent.

CASE 96 PES CAVUS

Examiner

Look at the patient's foot and examine him for relevant physical signs.

Locally

- Note the high arched foot.
- Perform a full neurological examination of the lower limbs, including testing for ataxia and for sensory and motor deficits.

Elsewhere

- Look for features of syringomyelia (e.g. wasting and trophic lesions of the hands with dissociated sensory loss and upper motor neurone signs in the lower limbs).
- Look for features of Friedreich's ataxia, e.g. ataxia, intention tremor, dysarthria, nystagmus (spinocerebellar tract), impaired joint and vibration sensation (posterior column), extensor plantar reflexes (corticospinal tracts), and optic atrophy. Absent ankle jerk with extensor plantar reflexes may be the sole manifestation. In peroneal muscle atrophy the legs look like inverted champagne bottles (see Case 97).

Candidate

This patient has pes cavus of the feet and ... (list all the signs you have found); put together, the pes cavus constitutes a manifestation of (give whatever your diagnosis is). If you have not reached a diagnosis just give your physical findings. It may well be that pes cavus is the only physical finding.

Examiner

What clinical conditions are associated with pes cavus?

Candidate

1. Friedreich's ataxia.
2. Peroneal muscular atrophy.
3. Syringomyelia.
4. Spina bifida.

Discussion on pes cavus

The intrinsic muscles of the sole of the foot run along the longitudinal arch of the foot. The short muscles of the foot are particularly responsible for the maintenance of the arch and any dysfunction of these muscles may be associated with a deformity such as pes cavus. The transverse arch of the foot is maintained by the transverse head of the adductor hallucis and by its oblique head. Increased height of the longitudinal arch commonly associated with dorsal contracture of the metatarsophalangeal joints results in pes cavus. In most cases, pes cavus is not associated with other neurological conditions but an association is present with Freidreich's ataxia, peroneal muscular atropy, syringomyelia and spina bifida.

CASE 97 CHARCOT–MARIE–TOOTH DISEASE

Examiner

Examine the patient's legs neurologically.

Locally

- Perform a complete neurological examination.
- Note the atrophy in the distal aspect of the thigh resulting in so-called 'inverted champagne bottle' shape of the legs.
- Note the atrophy of the peronie muscles, small muscles of the feet, long toe extensors and ankle dorsiflexors.
- Tendon reflexes are either diminished or absent in these wasted muscles.
- Sense of touch, pressure and joint position and vibration sensations are usually mildly affected in the lower limbs.
- Pes cavus may be present.
- Ask the patient to walk (gait abnormalities may be present).
- Look at the hands since they may be affected (claw hands).

Candidate

This patient has ... (give all your findings) which taken together are suggestive of Charcot–Marie–Tooth disease.

Examiner

Who was Charcot?

Candidate

He was a French physician and neurologist in the middle of the last century.

Examiner

What two investigations will help make a diagnosis?

Candidate

1. Nerve conduction studies.
2. Muscle biopsy.

Discussion on Charcot–Marie–Tooth disease

Hereditary neuropathies are characterized by a progressive form of neuropathy that may involve the motor neurones (motor neuropathy), sensory neurones (sensory neuropathy) or both the motor as well as sensory neurones (motor and sensory neuropathies). Clinical features may include pain, loss of sensation, gait disturbance and autonomic dysfunction. Charcot–Marie–Tooth disease is a relatively common hereditary disorder characterized by weakness and atrophy, primarily of the peroneal muscles due to segmental demyelination of peripheral nerves and associated degeneration of axons and anterior horn cells. Usually the condition is inherited as an autosomal dominant trait. Commonly, these patients are used for 'long cases' but sometimes they may be presented as short cases in the MRCP examination.

PART 9

Dermatology

GENERAL ADVICE

Common conditions used in the short cases include psoriasis; acanthosis nigricans; vitiligo; and erythema nodosum (see Case 97). Sometimes the skin manifestations of diabetes may be shown (necrobiosis; granuloma annulare; gangrene). Other skin conditions may include pityriasis versicolor; striae of Cushing's disease; alopecia; pyoderma gangrenosum.

CASE 98 PSORIASIS

Examiner

Look at this patient's leg/thigh/other.

Locally

- Note the number and site of skin lesions. They are usually on the extensor aspects.
- Describe them: usually well circumscribed skin macules, which become covered with fine silvery scales.
- Rub the lesions and allow the scales to drop off and then note the numerous small bleeding points to the dermis.

Elsewhere

- Look at the nails for any pitting, brittleness or irregular erosion (onycholysis).
- Sometimes an arthropathy of the terminal interphalangeal joints may be seen as well; if so the nails will always be affected.

Candidate

This patient has two (or whatever number) of skin lesions on the extensor aspect of the ... (go on to describe the site and the lesions themselves. Give any other physical signs). These features suggest a diagnosis of psoriasis.

Examiner

What factors exacerbate this condition?

Candidate

1. Local trauma (Koebner phenomenon).
2. Sunburn.
3. Topical skin medication.
4. Chloroquine therapy.
5. Systemic infections.

Examiner

What treatments are available?

Candidate

The condition can be brought under some degree of control
by the use of several topical and systemic therapies but there
is no permanent cure. Examples of some medications available
are:

1. Tar ointments.
2. Dithranol.
3. Topical steroids.
4. PUVA.
5. Cytotoxics like methotrexate.

Discussion on psoriasis

Psoriasis is a genetically determined condition that is characterized by well defined papules and erythematous plaques
covered by thickened scales. In most cases, the onset of these
lesions is seen in early adult life. Lesions are most commonly
noted on the extensor surface of the limbs (elbows and knees);
scalp, nails and other body areas (palms, soles, trunk) may
also be involved; arthritis may be seen in up to 20% cases. With
cutaneous trauma new lesions may appear (Koebner's phenomenon). Extensive involvement of the skin may result in
exfoliative erythroderma with disturbed control of body
temperature.

Excessive exfoliation may even lead to loss of protein, iron
and folate. The term 'guttate psoriasis' is used when psoriatic
areas are seen all over the body, usually after a few weeks of
streptococcal sore throat. 'Pustular psoriasis' is characterized
by the presence of numerous sterile pustules, an acute episode
of fever, chills, leucocytosis, hypocalcaemia and hypoalbuminaemia. This form of psoriasis requires urgent treatment.

CASE 99 ACANTHOSIS NIGRICANS

Examiner

Look at this patient's axillae/neck.

Locally

- The thickened, dark brown pigmented patches over the skin, usually bilateral and common in the axillae.

Elsewhere

- Look for similar patches on the neck and umbilical area.
- Look for evidence of carcinoma of the stomach, bowel or lung (an association is seen in 50% of cases).

Candidate

This patient has skin lesions suggestive of acanthosis nigricans. No clinical evidence of an underlying malignancy is present (or give findings if you have detected them).

Examiner

What malignancies in particular would you like to rule out?

Candidate

1. Carcinoma of the stomach.
2. Carcinoma of the bowel.
3. Carcinoma of the lung.

Examiner

What are other cutaneous manifestations of visceral malignancies?

Candidate

1. Thrombophlebitis migrans.
2. Dermatomyositis.
3. Ichthyosis (acquired).
4. Amyloid deposition.

Discussion on acanthosis nigricans

Acanthosis nigricans is characterized by the presence of symmetrical, soft brown hyperpigmented skin lesions, most commonly in the axillae, neck, pubis or umbilical area. In all cases, particularly if skin lesions appear in the middle years of life, all attempts must be made to exclude an underlying malignancy. Commonly associated tumours include carcinoma of the GIT (most commonly the stomach), uterus, ovary, prostate, breast and lung. In some cases the skin lesions may even appear months or years before the malignancy.

Although the exact cause of the skin lesions remains unclear, it is thought that the malignant tumour itself secretes some type of substance that causes the cutaneous changes of acanthosis nigricans. Removal of the tumour has been noted to result in regression of skin changes. Endocrine disorders including Cushing's disease, acromegaly, diabetes mellitus, hypothyroidism and hyperthyroidism may also be associated with acanthosis nigricans.

CASE 100 VITILIGO

Examiner

Look at the patient and examine appropriately.

Locally

• The skin vitiligo patches (hypopigmented lesions) will be obvious.
• Note the number and site of lesions (usually on sunlight exposed areas).

Elsewhere

• Look for evidence of pernicious anaemia, hyperthyroidism, Addison's disease and diabetes mellitus.

Candidate

This patient has vitiligo affecting . . . (give your findings and also mention whether there are obvious features of the autoimmune diseases mentioned or not).

Examiner

What other diseases are associated with vitiligo?

Candidate

Vitiligo is idiopathic in many cases and itself is thought to have an autoimmune basis. It is often associated with autoimmune diseases such as pernicious anaemia, hyperthyroidism, Addison's disease, and diabetes mellitus.

Examiner

What immunological investigations would you request?

Candidate

Auto-antibody screen, antibodies to thyroid, parietal cells, adrenals.

Examiner

What treatment would you consider?

Candidate

No satisfactory treatment exists at present. Cosmetic creams, protection from sunlight and oral and systemic psoralens have been prescribed with satisfactory results in about one third of patients.

Discussion on vitiligo

Vitiligo, which is characterized by patches of skin hypopigmentation, is commonly seen in areas of sunlight exposure and around body orifices and bony prominences (face, dorsal aspects of hands, mouth, eyes, nose, elbows, knees and genitals). The hair in the affected skin areas may become white.

The condition has an autoimmune basis. Circulating complement binding anti-melanocyte antibodies are commonly present. The course of the disease is unpredictable. Areas of repigmentation may appear as interrupted macules especially around the hair follicles. Rarely, leucoderma or hypopigmented skin areas may also develop as a result of the damage to the melanocytes by chemical toxins. A history of exposure to such chemicals is essential for diagnosis. When the hypopigmented areas occur because of leprosy (Hansen's disease), patients usually have hypoaesthesiae in the centre of the skin lesion and usually other peripheal nerves (ulnar, greater auricular, or peroneal, etc.) are thickened and can be palpated.

Index